PRACTICAL ASPECTS OF OPHTHALMIC OPTICS

PRACTICAL ASPECTS OF OPHTHALMIC OPTICS

Third Edition

Margaret Dowaliby, O.D.
Professor, Professional Studies
Southern California College of Optometry

Butterworth-Heinemann
Boston Oxford Melbourne Singapore Toronto Munich New Delhi Tokyo

Recognizing the importance of preserving what has been written, Butterworth–Heinemann prints its books on acid-free paper whenever possible.

Library of Congress Cataloging-in-Publication Data

Dowaliby, Margaret.
  Practical aspects of ophthalmic optics.

  Bibliography: p.
  Includes index.
  1. Optometry. 2. Optics, Physiological. I. Title.
[DNLM: 1. Eyeglasses. 2. Optometry. WW 352 D744p]
RE951.D68   1988   617.7'5   88-9955
ISBN 0-7506-9661-3 (previously ISBN 0-87873-081-8)

Butterworth–Heinemann
313 Washington Street
Newton, MA 02158–1626

10 9 8 7 6 5 4 3

Printed in the United States of America

To my mother, Hend

CONTENTS

ACKNOWLEDGMENTS

The material in this book is the second update from the original *Practical Aspects of Ophthalmic Optics* published almost two decades ago. I wish to extend special thanks to the experts in the optical field who helped verify certain sections; former president Jim Hull and Bob Strohbehn of Bartley Optical, Daniel A. Boucher of Younger Optics, Janet Martins, Roy Hinkemeyer, and Mike Jacobson of Vision-Ease, Greg Westmoreland of Titmus Optical, and Michael Randy Dowaliby, dispensing optician, Beverly Hills, California.

I want to express gratitude to Frank Brazelton, O.D.; Walter Chase, O.D.; William Brisbane, O.D.; faculty members of the Southern California College of Optometry, who gave invaluable expertise pertaining to their specialties; and Patricia Carlson, M.S.L.S., who researched the bibliography.

Particular thanks are extended to Judith Badstuebner and Patricia Humpres for their kindness in managing time and facilities to meet the completion date.

PREFACE

Eyecare as it is known today, with all the possibilities involved in providing visual efficiency, is to a large degree the result of tremendous strides made in the field of ophthalmic optics. Advances in the design of conventional ophthalmic lenses have resulted in an optical efficiency that until recently was within the realm of improbability. Progress in the area of unusual lens design has made it possible for many patients to enjoy visual corrections that previously presented optical and cosmetic problems.

By classic definition, ophthalmic optics is that aspect of geometric and physical optics dealing with the application of lenses to the human eye. The contemporary field of ophthalmic optics involves itself with designs of lenses mounted in frames (eyewear), lenses worn within the conjunctival sac (contact lenses), and lenses worn as magnifying units (low-vision aids). Each of these types of visual correction has undergone dramatic improvement in the past decade. To explain the advancements fully, books need to be devoted to each area. This volume concerns itself solely with lenses mounted into conventional eyeframes. It is highly practical in nature and involves itself with the optics of today's wide range of lens designs. Some lenses are simple, some complex, but each in its own way serves as the best possible visual aid for the care of a specific patient.

This area is of primary concern to most practitioners because the majority of patients seeking visual care are aided by a correction in the form of conventional eyewear. This book discusses the changes in single-vision lenses, the constantly expanding field of multifocal prescribing, the advances in the field of safety eyewear, the complexities in today's world of absorptive lenses, and the growing expansion of aids that make lenses optically superior as well as cosmetically pleasing.

This book's goals are to give the practitioner the opportunity to reevaluate the availability of optical products that best serve the patient and to acquaint the student with the practical aspects involved in the field of ophthalmic optics.

Chapter 1

CHARACTERISTICS OF LENSES

INTRODUCTION

An ophthalmic lens is a transparent medium bound by two polished surfaces, either plane or curved, that act as an optical system. Two substances are used in the production of lenses: glass, the most widely prescribed, and plastic, recommended with increasing frequency.

Modern ophthalmic lenses are prescribed for many reasons. Their primary use is the correction of refractive errors. They also may aid in correcting faulty binocular vision. They may act as protection against foreign objects. Some designs serve as absorptive lenses to filter those portions of the spectrum that prove uncomfortable or harmful to the patient.

Refractive errors result when light rays entering the eye do not focus on the retina. Basically three conditions exist: hyperopia, or far-sightedness; myopia, or near-sightedness; and astigmatism.

In cases of hyperopia, light rays entering the eye focus behind the retina and must be converged to provide clear, comfortable vision. This is accomplished by prescribing plus (convex) lenses, which exhibit the following characteristics:

1. A plus lens converges parallel light. If the light is converging as it passes through the lens, the convergence is increased; if it is diverging, either it diverges less or it may converge, depending upon the power of the lens.

2. Parallel rays of light passing through a plus lens will focus at a specific distance, depending upon the power of the lens.

3. The center thickness of a plus lens is greater than its edge thickness.

4. When the observer views an object through a plus lens, the image is magnified.

5. When a plus lens is held before the eye so that the secondary focal point falls behind the retina, a movement of the lens results in an opposite motion of objects viewed through the lens. This movement is technically referred to as "against motion."

6. The effective power of a plus lens increases as it is moved away from the eye.

In cases of myopia, light rays entering the eye focus in front of the retina. To correct this anomaly, minus lenses are prescribed. These concave lenses demonstrate the following characteristics:

1. Minus lenses diverge parallel light. If the light is diverging as it passes through the lens, the divergence increases; if converging, it will converge less or diverge, depending upon the power of the lens.

2. Light incident upon a minus lens will not come to a point focus.

3. Objects viewed through a concave lens are minified.

4. The edge thickness of a minus lens is greater than its center thickness.

5. When a minus lens is held before the eye, the object viewed moves in the same direction as the movement of the lens. This technically is referred to as "with motion."

6. The effective power of a minus lens decreases as it is moved away from the eye.

In cases of astigmatism, light rays entering the eye are not focused at a single point but instead focus as two line images at right angles to each other. This anomaly, known as regular astigmatism, requires a correcting lens with power that gradually increases from a minimum in one meridian to the maximum amount in the meridian 90° away. These are known as the principal meridians of the lens and coincide with the major meridians of the eye. The correcting lenses for regular astigmatism are known as cylinders and have the following characteristics:

1. A conventional cylindrical lens has one toric surface (a surface having meridians of least and greatest curvature located at right angles to each other).

2. The meridian of least power is known as the axis; the meridian of maximum power is 90° away. In this 90° span there is a gradual increase in the power of the cylinder, the amount dependent on the angle subtended from the axis.

3. When a line object is viewed through a cylinder so that the axis or the meridian of greatest power coincides with that line, rotation of the lens produces a "break" in its continuity. If the motion of the line is opposite to the movement of the lens, the meridian involved is the plus cylinder axis or the meridian of least plus power. Conversely, if the movement is in the same direction, the meridian is the minus cylinder axis or the meridian of most plus power.

Note: There is another type of astigmatism, relatively rare and known as irregular astigmatism, where the two principal meridians of the eye are not 90° apart. Cylindrical lenses cannot fully correct this anomaly.

DESIGNATION OF LENS POWER

The basic unit of power for lenses is the diopter, usually abbreviated as "D." By definition, the number of diopters of power is equal to the reciprocal of the focal length of the lens in meters. Therefore, the formula for dioptric power is stated as follows:

$$1/\text{focal length (meters)} = \text{diopters}$$

Example:

If the focal length of a lens is 1 meter, then $1/1\text{m} = 1.00\text{D}$. If the focal length is 40 centimeters, then $1/.4\text{m} = 2.50\text{D}$.

Conversely, the focal length of a lens can be found by taking the reciprocal of its dioptric power:

$$1/\text{diopters} = \text{focal length (meters)}$$

Example:

If the lens power is +3.00 diopters, then 1/3.00D = 33.3 centimeters.
If the lens power is +0.25 diopters, then 1/0.25D = 4 meters.
Note: Focal length is measured from the *back* surface of the lens to the point of focus. This interval is known as the vertex focal distance. Therefore, the stated dioptric power of an ophthalmic lens is actually the vertex power.

POWER OF LENSES

Ophthalmic lenses are manufactured in 1/8D intervals. This difference has been found to be the smallest increment discernible to the patient, although quarter diopter steps present a degree of accuracy sufficient in most cases. Thus, the available dioptric range of ophthalmic lenses includes plano (no power, but possessing the quality optical characteristics), +0.12D, +0.25D, +0.37D, +0.50D, +0.62D, +0.75D, +0.87D, +1.00D, +1.12D, +1.25D, etc.; and −0.12D, −0.25D, −0.37D, etc.

OTHER LENS CLASSIFICATIONS

Spherical Lenses

Ophthalmic lenses are also classified as spheres, plano-cylinders, and sphero-cylinders (combination of sphere and cylinder).

Spherical lenses are designated as such because their curved surfaces are similar to sections of a sphere. The same refractive power is found in all meridians and, depending on the prescription, the lens may converge light (plus or convex lenses), diverge light (minus or concave lenses), or leave parallel rays unaltered (plano lenses).

Plano-cylindrical Lenses

A plano-cylindrical lens has one meridian that contains no power; it is known as the axis and is the reference meridian of all cylindrical lenses. Ninety degrees away from the axis is the toroidal meridian of maximum power. In the other meridians, the cylinder power varies between the axis and the meridian of maximum curvature according to the following formula:

$$F' = F_{\text{total cylinder}} \times \sin^2 \theta$$
F' = cylinder power of any given meridian
$F_{\text{total cylinder}}$ = total power of the cylinder
θ = angle between the axis and the meridian in question

The powers of five meridians in a plano-cylindrical lens are easily calculated, and by knowing these it is possible to estimate rather accurately the power in any other meridian. Applying the formula $F' = F (\sin^2 \theta)$, the power 30° away from the axis is equal to ¼ of the total power of the cylinder; 45° away, ½ the power; and 60° away, ¾ of the total cylindrical power.

The simplicity of computing the powers in the meridians mentioned is illustrated by the following examples:

PROBLEM:

Given a $-2.00 \times 30°$ lens, find the power in the following meridians: (a) 180°, (b) 30°, (c) 60°, (d) 90°, (e) 120°.

SOLUTION:

$F' = F (\sin^2 \theta)$
(a) $F' = (-2.00) (\sin^2 30°) = (-2.00) (0.25) = -0.50D$
(b) $F' = (-2.00) (\sin^2 \theta) = (-2.00) (0.00) = -0.00D$
(c) $F' = (-2.00) (\sin^2 30°) = (-2.00) (0.25) = -0.50D$
(d) $F' = (-2.00) (\sin^2 60°) = (-2.00) (0.75) = -1.50D$
(e) $F' = (-2.00) (\sin^2 90°) = (-2.00) (1.00) = -2.00D$

PROBLEM:

Given a plano + 1.00 cylindrical lens with axis 90°, compute the powers in the following meridians: (a) 90°, (b) 60°, (c) 45°, (d) 30°, (e) 180°.

SOLUTION:

(a) Plano at 90° (no power at axis)
(b) +0.25D at 60° (¼ of +1.00D, 30° from axis)
(c) +0.50D at 45° (½ of +1.00D, 45° from axis)
(d) +0.75D at 30° (¾ of +1.00D, 60° from axis)
(e) +1.00D at 180° (total power 90° from axis)

If accurate power in meridians not 30°, 45°, 60°, or 90° from the axis is desired, it is necessary to utilize the formula given: $F' = F (\sin^2 \theta)$.

PROBLEM:

Given a $-1.00 \times 180°$ lens, find the power in the following meridians: (a) 180°, (b) 5°, (c) 15°, (d) 25°, (e) 30°, (f) 40°, (g) 45°, (h) 55°, (i) 60°, (j) 70°, (k) 80°, (l) 90°.

SOLUTION:

$F' = F (\sin^2 \theta)$
(a) $F' = (-1.00) (\sin^2 0°) = (-1.00) (0.00) = 0.00D$
(b) $F' = (-1.00) (\sin^2 5°) = (-1.00) (0.01) = -0.01D$
(c) $F' = (-1.00) (\sin^2 15°) = (-1.00) (0.07) = -0.07D$
(d) $F' = (-1.00) (\sin^2 25°) = (-1.00) (0.18) = -0.18D$
(e) $F' = (-1.00) (\sin^2 30°) = (-1.00) (0.25) = -0.25D$
(f) $F' = (-1.00) (\sin^2 40°) = (-1.00) (0.41) = -0.41D$
(g) $F' = (-1.00) (\sin^2 45°) = (-1.00) (0.50) = -0.50D$
(h) $F' = (-1.00) (\sin^2 55°) = (-1.00) (0.67) = -0.67D$
(i) $F' = (-1.00) (\sin^2 60°) = (-1.00) (0.75) = -0.75D$
(j) $F' = (-1.00) (\sin^2 70°) = (-1.00) (0.88) = -0.88D$
(k) $F' = (-1.00) (\sin^2 80°) = (-1.00) (0.97) = -0.97D$
(l) $F' = (-1.00) (\sin^2 90°) = (-1.00) (1.00) = -1.00D$

Sphero-cylindrical Lenses

Sphero-cylindrical lenses have a spherical component that is found throughout the lens. To determine the total power in a particular meridian, the cylinder is computed in the manner previously discussed and added to the sphere.

PROBLEM:

Given a $+3.00 + 1.00 \times 90°$ lens, find the power in the following meridians: (a) 90°, (b) 60°, (c) 45°, (d) 30°, (e) 180°.

SOLUTION:

$F' = F_{sphere} + F_{cylinder} (\sin^2 \theta)$
(a) $F' = +3.00 + (+1.00) (\sin^2 0°) = +3.00D$
(b) $F' = +3.00 + (+1.00) (\sin^2 30°) = +3.25D$
(c) $F' = +3.00 + (+1.00) (\sin^2 45°) = +3.50D$
(d) $F' = +3.00 + (+1.00) (\sin^2 60°) = +3.75D$
(e) $F' = +3.00 + (+1.00) (\sin^2 90°) = +4.00D$

PROBLEM:

Given a $+3.00 - 3.00 \times 60°$ lens, find the power in the following meridians: (a) 60°, (b) 90°, (c) 105°, (d) 120°, (e) 150°.

SOLUTION:

$F' = F_{sphere} + F_{cylinder} (\sin^2 \theta)$
(a) $F' = +3.00 + (-3.00) (\sin^2 0°)$
$= +3.00 + (-3.00) (0.00) = +3.00D$
(b) $F' = +3.00 + (-3.00) (\sin^2 30°)$
$= +3.00 + (-3.00) (0.25) = +2.25D$
(c) $F' = +3.00 + (-3.00) (\sin^2 45°)$
$= +3.00 + (-3.00) (0.50) = +1.50D$
(d) $F' = +3.00 + (-3.00) (\sin^2 60°)$
$= +3.00 + (-3.00) (0.75) = +0.75D$
(e) $F' = +3.00 + (-3.00) (\sin^2 90°)$
$= +3.00 + (-3.00) (1.00) = +0.00D$

PROBLEM:

Given a $-4.00 - 1.00 \times 180°$ lens, find the power in the following meridians: (a) 180°, (b) 30°, (c) 45°, (d) 60°, (e) 90°.

SOLUTION:

$F' = F_{sphere} + F_{cylinder} (\sin^2 \theta)$
(a) $F' = -4.00 + (-1.00) (\sin^2 0°)$
$= -4.00 + (-1.00) (0.00) = -4.00D$
(b) $F' = -4.00 + (-1.00) (\sin^2 30°)$
$= -4.00 + (-1.00) (0.25) = -4.25D$
(c) $F' = -4.00 + (-1.00) (\sin^2 45°)$
$= -4.00 + (-1.00) (0.50) = -4.50D$
(d) $F' = -4.00 + (-1.00) (\sin^2 60°)$
$= -4.00 + (-1.00) (0.75) = -4.75D$
(e) $F' = -4.00 + (-1.00) (\sin^2 90°)$
$= -4.00 + (-1.00) (1.00) = -5.00D$

The cylinder power of a plano-cylinder or sphero-cylinder lens can be ground on either the convex or concave surface, but most manufacturers are phasing out plus cylinder lenses because minus designs keep meridional magnification at a minimum.

In cases of high-power cylinder prescriptions, minus cylinders offer a definite cosmetic advantage. Since the changes in curvature to accommodate the cylinder are on the back surface, the thickness difference is not as apparent when the glasses are worn.

The cylinder form of a multifocal lens is predetermined by the design, and the cylindrical surface is always on the side opposite the segment.

WRITING THE PRESCRIPTION

An ophthalmic prescription is correctly written to two decimal places. If less than 1 diopter of power is involved, it is customary in some areas to precede the decimal point with a zero. For example, a quarter-diopter of power could be written as 0.25D.

The spherical power is first noted, sometimes followed by the diopters of sphere (D.S.). The next quotation is the cylinder, which may be affixed to the diopters of cylinder (D.C.). The axis is preceded by a multiplication sign and is sometimes followed by a degree sign. For example:

$$+2.00 \text{ D.S.} - 3.00 \text{ D.C.} \times 90°$$

However, for simplicity, when writing the prescription, it is customary to omit D.S., D.C., and the degree sign. The prescription then reads as follows:

$$+2.00 - 3.00 \times 90$$

It is usually best to eliminate the degree sign because it can be mistaken for a zero. For example, note that the prescription $+1.00 + 4.25 \times 10°$ could be mistaken for $+1.00 + 4.25 \times 100$ if the degree sign were not in correct proportion to the other numbers.

TRANSPOSITION

Practitioners usually write the prescription in the same cylinder form they used when examining the patient with the refractor. However, because most laboratories now use minus-cylinder, single-vision lenses and multifocals have a predetermined cylinder form, it may be necessary to convert the written prescription from plus to minus cylinders (or vice versa) without actually changing the lens power. This conversion is known as "transposition." Plano-cylinder and sphero-cylinder lenses are transposed by the following method:

1. Add the powers of the sphere and cylinder algebraically. If the lens is a plano-cylinder, the sphere power is noted as zero.

2. Change the sign of the cylinder retaining the same amount of cylinder.

3. Add or subtract 90°, whichever leaves the axis 180° or less.

Sometimes the principal meridians of the eye are refracted using spherical lenses. This may be necessary when trial lens examinations are performed (i.e., for small children, "home refractions" for invalids, etc.). The prescription may originally be recorded as two crossed cylinders with the axes positioned 90° apart. For example, if +1.00D neutralizes the horizontal meridian of the eye and +3.00D neutralizes the vertical, the result is +1.00 × 90° ◯ + 3.00 × 180°. The crossed-cylinder prescription is then transposed into sphero-cylinder form.

The following is the procedure for transposing into plus cylinder form:

1. Transpose the lowest plus cylinder so that both axes are the same.

$$+1.00 \times 90° \text{ becomes } + 1.00 - 1.00 \times 180°$$

2. Algebraically add the transposed +1.00 − 1.00 × 180° to the remaining plano-cylinder retaining the same axis:

$$\begin{array}{r} +1.00 - 1.00 \times 180° \\ + 3.00 \times 180° \\ \hline +1.00 + 2.00 \times 180° \end{array}$$

To transpose into minus cylinder form, transpose +1.00 + 2.00 × 180° into +3.00 − 2.00 × 90° by the procedure outlined earlier in this chapter.

A sphero-cylinder prescription can be changed to cross-cylinders 90° to each other. The following problem shows the procedure.

PROBLEM:

Transpose +1.00 + 2.00 × 180° into cross-cylinder form.

PROCEDURE:

1. Record the sphere as a cylinder, axis 90° away from the original:

$$+1.00 \times 90°$$

2. Add the original sphere and cylinder algebraically and record as a cylinder at the original axis:

$$+3.00 \times 180°$$

3. Combine the answers for (1) and (2).

SOLUTION:

$+1.00 \times 90° \circlearrowright + 3.00 \times 180°$

COMBINING TWO CROSS CYLINDERS THAT ARE NOT 90° APART

It is extremely rare, but possible, for a prescription to be written with the cylinders not positioned 90° apart. The prescription needs to be rewritten in sphero-cylinder form before the lens can be manufactured. There are two methods by which this can be accomplished. One is a graphic procedure; the other is a formula method. Two examples of each are given.

PROBLEM I:

What is the plus sphero-cylinder equivalent of the following prescription?

$$+3.00 \times 55° \circlearrowright + 1.00 \times 50°$$

GRAPHIC PROCEDURE:

1. The cylinder powers are graphed along an "A" line and a "B" line. The "A" cylinder has the axis closest to the numerical value zero.

    "A" cylinder = $+1.00 \times 50°$
    "B" cylinder = $+3.00 \times 55°$

2. "A" cylinder is plotted on the base line. "B" cylinder is plotted 2α degrees away. α is the difference between the two axes (55° − 50°); in this case $\alpha = 5°$.

    $$2\alpha = 10°$$

3. Graph cylinder "A" and cylinder "B," and complete the parallelogram by drawing a dotted line from the point of origin to the opposite extremity of the parallelogram (Figure 1.1).

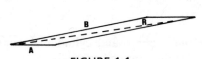

FIGURE 1.1

4. The dotted line "R" represents the resultant cylinder, and "R" measured = $+4.00D$.

5. The new sphere (S) is determined using the formula

$$S = \frac{A_{cyl} + B_{cyl} - R_{cyl}}{2}$$

$$S = \frac{+1.00 + 3.00 - 4.00}{2}$$

$$= 0.00D$$

6. The new axis is the axis of "A" cylinder plus γ. The angle between "A" and "R" is 2γ (measured 8°).

$$\gamma = 4°.$$

The new axis is 54° (50° + 4°).

GRAPHIC SOLUTION TO PROBLEM I:

Plus sphero-cylinder equivalent = plano + 4.00 × 54°

FORMULA PROCEDURE:

To solve a cross-cylinder problem by the formula method, the following trigonometric functions need to be considered:
In the first quadrant all functions are positive.

In the second quadrant the sine only is positive.

In the third quadrant the tangent only is positive.

In the fourth quadrant the cosine only is positive.

1. The formula for the resultant cylinder is

$$R_{cyl} = \sqrt{A^2 + B^2 + 2AB \cos 2\alpha}$$

If 2α is less than 90°, the formula stays as above. If 2α is exactly 90°, the term $2AB \cos 2\alpha$ drops and the formula reads $R_{cyl} = \sqrt{A^2 + B^2}$ (because $\cos 90° = 0$). If 2α is more than 90°, the cosine term becomes negative (cosine is negative in the second quadrant). The formula now reads:

$$R_{cyl} = \sqrt{A^2 + B^2 - 2AB \cos 2\alpha}$$

In this problem the first formula applies because 2α is less than 90°.

$$R_{cyl} = \sqrt{A^2 + B^2 + 2AB \cos 2\alpha}$$
$$= \sqrt{1^2 + 3^2 + 2(1)(3) \cos 10°}$$
$$= \sqrt{15.91}$$
$$= +3.99D$$

2. The sphere is determined by the formula

$$S = \frac{A_{cyl} + B_{cyl} - R_{cyl}}{2}$$

$$= \frac{+1.00 + 3.00 - 3.99}{2}$$

$$= +0.005D$$

3. The new axis is determined by the formula "A" axis + γ, and γ is found using the formula

$$\frac{\sin 2\gamma}{B_{cyl}} = \frac{\sin 2\alpha}{R_{cyl}}$$

$$\frac{\sin 2\gamma}{+3.00} = \frac{\sin 10°}{+3.99}$$

$$\sin 2\gamma = \frac{+3.00\,(0.17365)}{+3.99}$$

$$2\gamma = 8°$$

$$\gamma = 4°$$

4. The axis of "A" + γ = 50° + 4° = 54°.

FORMULA SOLUTION TO PROBLEM I:

Plus cylinder form prescription = +0.005 + 3.99 × 54°

PROBLEM II:

Change the following prescription into plus sphero-cylinder form.

$$+3.00 \times 60°\,\supset\, - 4.00 \times 25°$$

GRAPHIC PROCEDURE:

1. Transpose both cylinders to plus cylinder form. Note: Before graphing, cylinders need to be the same sign. Transposed, the formula reads:

$$+3.00 \times 60°\,\supset\, - 4.00 + 4.00 \times 115°$$

2. The two cylinders are +3.00 × 60° $\supset$ + 4.00 × 115°. The "A" cylinder = +3.00D (numerical value closest to zero). The "B" cylinder = +4.00D.

$$\alpha = 115° - 60° = 55°$$

$$2\alpha = 110°$$

3. Graph cylinder "A" and cylinder "B" and complete the parallelogram (Figure 1.2).

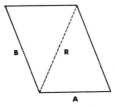

FIGURE 1.2

4. The resultant cylinder "R" measures +4.10D.

5. Determine the new sphere:

$$S = \frac{A_{cyl} + B_{cyl} - R_{cyl}}{2} + \text{original sphere (after transposition)}$$

$$= \frac{+3.00 + 4.00 - 4.10}{2} + (-4.00)$$

$$= -2.55D$$

6. The new axis is equal to "A" axis + γ.

$$2\gamma = 66°$$
$$\gamma = 33°$$

The new axis is equal to $60° + 33° = 93°$.

GRAPHIC SOLUTION TO PROBLEM II:

Plus cylinder prescription $= -2.55 + 4.10 \times 93°$

FORMULA PROCEDURE:

1. Transpose so that both cylinders are in plus-cylinder form, $+3.00 \times 60° \subset -4.00 + 4.00 \times 115°$.

2. "A" cylinder $= +3.00 \times 60°$ (numerical value of axis closest to zero) "B" cylinder $= +4.00 \times 115°$

$$\alpha = 115° - 60° = 55°$$
$$2\alpha = 110°$$

3. The formula for the new cylinder is

$$R_{cyl} = \sqrt{A^2 + B^2 + 2AB \cos 2\alpha}$$
$$R_{cyl} = \sqrt{3^2 + 4^2 + 2(3)(4) \cos 110°}$$
$$= \sqrt{16.9}$$
$$= +4.11D$$

4. The new sphere is determined by

$$S = \frac{A_{cyl} + B_{cyl} - R_{cyl}}{2} + \text{original sphere}$$

$$S = \frac{+3.00 + 4.00 - 4.11}{2} + (-4.00)$$

$$= -2.56D$$

5. Determine the new axis by the formula "A" axis $+ \gamma$, where γ is calculated using the formula

$$\frac{\sin 2\gamma}{B_{cyl}} = \frac{\sin 2\alpha}{R_{cyl}}$$

$$\frac{\sin 2\gamma}{+4.00} = \frac{\sin 110°}{+4.11}$$

$$2\gamma = 66°$$

$$\gamma = 33°$$

Therefore, the new axis is $60° + 33° = 93°$.

FORMULA SOLUTION TO PROBLEM II:

Plus cylinder prescription $= -2.56 + 4.11 \times 93°$

OPTICAL CROSS

An optical cross is a simple cross diagram indicating the powers in the various lens meridians. Intersecting lines 90° apart representing the axis and the meridian of maximum power are always included; other lines may be used to represent meridians of special interest.

Example:

Usually prescriptions are placed on an optical cross to determine quickly the power in a particular meridian (Figures 1.3 and 1.4).

Prescriptions are placed on an optical cross by the following method:

1. The spherical correction is noted in the principal meridians although it is understood to encompass the entire lens.
2. The cylindrical correction is noted 90° away from the axis.
3. The sphere and the cylinder are added algebraically in the meridian involved.

Example:

Note: It is customary to mark the powers in the upper quadrants of the cross (Figures 1.5 and 1.6), although it is understood that the entire meridian in question is involved.

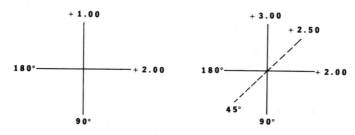

FIGURE 1.3   *+1.00 + 1.00 × 90°*   **FIGURE 1.4**   *+3.00 − 1.00 × 90°*

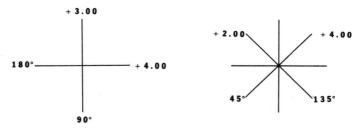

FIGURE 1.5   *+3.00 + 1.00 × 90°*   **FIGURE 1.6**   *+4.00 − 2.00 × 45°*

A prescription can be written three ways:

1.   In plus-cylinder form
2.   In minus-cylinder form
3.   In the cross-cylinder form

The following powers are noted on an optical cross (Figure 1.7).

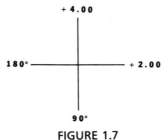

FIGURE 1.7

PROBLEM:

Write the prescription on this cross (Figure 1.7) in (a) plus-cylinder form, (b) minus-cylinder form, (c) cross-cylinder form.

SOLUTION:

(a) +2.00 + 2.00 × 180°
(b) +4.00 − 2.00 × 90°
(c) +2.00 × 90° ◯ + 4.00 × 180°

PROBLEM:

The following powers are noted on an optical cross (Figure 1.8). Write the prescription in the following three forms: (a) plus cylinder, (b) minus cylinder, (c) cross cylinder.

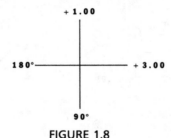

FIGURE 1.8

SOLUTION:

(a) +1.00 + 2.00 × 90°
(b) +3.00 − 2.00 × 180°
(c) +3.00 × 90° ◯ + 1.00 × 180°

POSITIONING THE CYLINDER

Cylinder meridians are designated from 0° to 180°. Viewed from the front surface (looking at the patient), meridians are noted counterclockwise

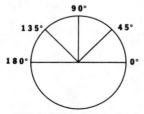

FIGURE 1.9   *Right lens*

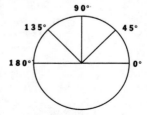

FIGURE 1.10   *Left lens*

(Figures 1.9 and 1.10) beginning with 0° at the patient's left and increasing to 180°.

BASE CURVES OF SPHERICAL LENSES

Ophthalmic lenses can be grouped according to base curves. When spherical lenses are involved, the base curve is the power of one surface common to a specific lens series. With toric lenses, it is the weakest curve on the cylindrical surface; with multifocals, the base curve is the spherical curve on the segment side. The reference surface in each instance usually guarantees a standardization that manufacturers accept as a basis for the design of lenses. However, when ordering, it is best to specify the curve on the spherical side of the lens. The base curve will identify a spherical single-vision lens with one of the five conventional lens forms.

1. Plano-convex or Plano-concave

The base curve of these lenses is a plane surface with the total lens power ground on the opposite side (Figures 1.11 and 1.12). Since the flattest curve of a lens is the ocular surface, the plano-convex lens has the total power ground on the nonocular side; the plano-concave lens has the total power on the ocular surface. Use of this form is limited to high-power prescriptions, although plano-convex and plano-concave lenses are sometimes found in older trial lens sets.

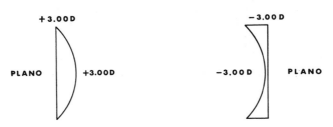

FIGURE 1.11   *Plano-convex*   FIGURE 1.12   *Plano-concave*

2. Biconvex and Biconcave

The biconvex lens features two convex surfaces usually of equal curvature (Figures 1.13 and 1.14). Similarly, the biconcave design has both surfaces usually of equal minus power. It is rare to have a biconvex or biconcave lens with different curvatures, but, when it does occur either surface may be considered the base curve. This lens form is rarely manufactured, except in trial lens sets and some low-vision aids.

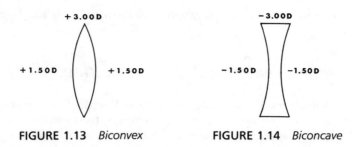

FIGURE 1.13 *Biconvex*   **FIGURE 1.14** *Biconcave*

3. Periscopic

The periscopic lens features a base curve of 1.25D. If the total lens power is plus, the base curve is −1.25D located on the ocular surface. With minus power lenses the base curve is +1.25D and is found on the nonocular side. The power of the opposite surface is the curve that, when combined with +1.25D or −1.25D (Figures 1.15 and 1.16), gives the total lens power. With the exception of certain high-power prescriptions, the periscopic lens is rarely used today.

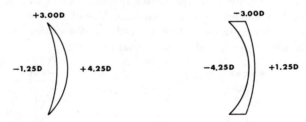

FIGURE 1.15 *Plus periscopic*   **FIGURE 1.16** *Minus periscopic*

4. Meniscus

By convention, meniscus lenses have a base curve of 6.00D. However, any lens not of plano, biconvex, biconcave, periscopic, or corrected-curve form can be considered a meniscus lens. If the total power is plus, the base curve is always the ocular surface. The outside curve is that which, when combined with −6.00D (Figure 1.17), will give the desired power. With minus power lenses, the base curve is a plus curvature (usually +6.00D) (Figure 1.18) located on the outside surface. The meniscus lens is manufactured by many optical companies and is widely used in filling prescriptions.

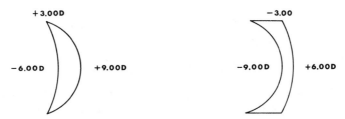

FIGURE 1.17 *Plus meniscus*   FIGURE 1.18 *Minus meniscus*

5. Corrected Curve

The base curve for each corrected lens varies according to the manufacturer, and the appropriate power chart needs to be consulted for specific values. While corrected lenses are designed to eliminate or reduce aberrations present in the peripheral portions of the lens, their importance is deemphasized with the fashion use of large-eye frames. It is impossible to eliminate peripheral distortion when oversize lenses are worn.

BASE CURVES OF CYLINDRICAL SINGLE-VISION LENSES

The base curve of a cylindrical lens is the weakest curve on the cylinder side. When the cylinder power is on the convex surface, the meridian having the least plus power is the base curve. For example, a lens +1.00 + 2.00 × 90° with an inside curve of −6.00D has a base curve of +7.00D. This becomes evident by illustrating a side view of the lens with a cross line noting the cylindrical surface (Figure 1.19). The curves are designated as follows:

1.   The power on the concave surface is marked −6.00D.

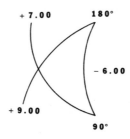

FIGURE 1.19

2.   On the convex surface, the power in the meridian of the axis is +7.00D. It is the power that, when combined algebraically with the ocular surface (−6.00D), yields the spherical component of the prescription. For example, +7.00D + (−6.00D) = +1.00D.

3.   The power of the curve 90° away from the axis is +9.00D. Because the axis is the meridian of least power, the cross curve manifests more plus power by the amount of the cylinder (i.e., +2.00D).

4.   Because by definition the base curve is the weakest curve on the cylinder side, the base curve is +7.00D (meridian of least power).

When the cylinder is on the concave surface, the meridian having the least power is the base curve. For example (Figure 1.20), a lens +1.00 − 3.00 × 180° with an outside curve of +7.00D has a base curve of −6.00D.

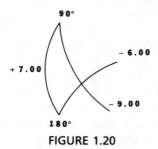

FIGURE 1.20

1.   The power on the convex surface is +7.00D.

2.   On the concave surface, the power in the meridian of the axis is −6.00D. When this power is combined algebraically with the nonocular surface (+7.00D), the result is the spherical component of the prescription, that is, +7.00D + (−6.00D) = +1.00D.

3.   The power at 90° is −9.00D (cylinder difference of 3.00D).

4.   The base curve is −6.00D (weakest curve on the cylinder side).

Note: Laboratories are also identifying the spherical outside curve of minus cylinder lenses as the base curve. Be specific when ordering.

VERTEX DISTANCE AND ITS RELATION TO EFFECTIVE POWER

Emmetropia is that condition in which distant objects are focused clearly on the retina without the use of accommodation. The far point of the emmetropic eye is at infinity; that is, rays of light from infinity are conjugate with the retina (20 feet or more is considered optical infinity).

If a patient is not emmetropic (hyperopic, myopic, or astigmatic), correcting lenses must be placed in a certain position to allow parallel light entering the eye to focus on the retina. By common consent, manufacturers calculate the optics of lenses so that the power is true when the back surface of a lens is 13.75mm anterior to the cornea (vertex power). In practice, this distance is rarely measured because the discrepancy of a few millimeters normally does not make a significant difference in visual acuity.

However, when a high-power prescription is involved, vertex distance is critical and should be measured to determine the "effective power" of the lens. Effective power is defined as the vergence power of an optical system with respect to a particular reference point other than the principal point. In practice, the retina of the eye is usually designated as the reference plane and lens effectivity determined accordingly. The primary concern is alteration in effectivity when a high-power lens is moved closer to or further from the eye (i.e., as the vertex distance is changed). Moving a convex lens away from the eye increases its effective power because the image is now formed in front of the retina; consequently, a weaker plus lens may have to be prescribed. Conversely, moving a concave lens away from the eye reduces its effectivity since the image is now theoretically formed behind the retina.

The change in effectivity as the vertex distance is altered is calculated by the following formula:

$$F_{\text{effective power}} = \frac{F_{\text{true power}}}{1 - dF_{\text{true power}}}$$

$F_{\text{true power}}$ refers to the actual power of the lens as determined by the focal length; $F_{\text{effective power}}$ refers to the lens power with respect to the retina (the reference plane). The distance in meters that the lens is moved from its original position is indicated by the letter d.

PROBLEM:

A + 10.00D lens that forms a clear image on the retina is moved 5 mm further from the eye. Compute the effective power in this new position.

SOLUTION:

$$F_{\text{effective power}} = \frac{F_{\text{true power}}}{1 - dF_{\text{true power}}}$$

$$= \frac{+10.00}{1 - (0.005)(10)}$$

$$= +10.53D$$

PROBLEM:

A patient is refracted 10mm anterior to his corneal vertex. He is found to need a $-10.00D$ lens in front of each eye. If his glasses are worn 15mm anterior to the corneal vertex, what is the effective power in this position?

SOLUTION:

$$F_{\text{eff}} = \frac{F_{\text{true}}}{1 - dF_{\text{true}}}$$

$$= \frac{-10.00}{1 - (0.005)(-10)}$$

$$= -9.50D$$

ABERRATIONS OF LENSES

Lens aberrations result when rays from a point source fail to form a perfect point image after traversing an optical system. All ophthalmic lenses have certain aberrations. One, chromatic aberration, derives from the nature of glass; the other five—spherical aberration, coma, marginal or oblique astigmatism, curvature of field, and distortion—are a result of the lens design. Some of these aberrations may be reduced; in essence, this is the purpose of corrected-curve lenses. However, it is important to recognize that the increased use of oversize blanks must invalidate some of the applications of corrected-curve lenses.

1. Chromatic Aberration

Chromatic aberration results from the splitting of white light into component spectral colors when it is refracted by a glass lens (Figure 1.21). Because each wavelength has a different speed in any medium heavier than air, glass has a different refractive index for the various wavelengths.

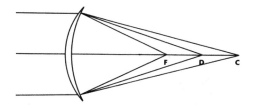

FIGURE 1.21   *Chromatic aberration*

This dispersive property manifests itself by focusing the blue, or "F," line of the spectrum before the yellow, or "D," line; the red of the "C" line focuses after the "D."

Note: The power of a lens is arbitrarily determined by the focus of the "D" (yellow) line of the Fraunhofer spectrum. These lines denote particular colors of the spectrum, each occupying a constant position corresponding to a specific wavelength.

Although chromatic aberration can be corrected by combining two thin lenses of different indices to obtain an achromatic doublet, this aberration is not considered serious. Single-vision lenses manufactured of crown glass have a relatively low dispersive value. Also, the eye itself is not achromatic.

2. Spherical Aberration

Spherical aberration results because different zones of a lens have different powers (Figure 1.22). Peripheral and paraxial rays focus at different points along the axis, but because the pupil acts to limit the number of rays entering the eye, spherical aberration is not an ophthalmic problem.

3. Coma

Coma occurs because different areas of a lens project images of different size (Figure 1.23). An image of a point off the optical axis appears comet-shaped with the tail pointing toward the axis. Coma is not a concern in ophthalmic lenses because the pupil acts as an aperture to eliminate the peripheral rays.

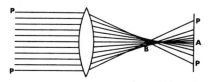

FIGURE 1.22   *Spherical aberration*

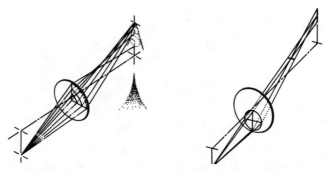

FIGURE 1.23 *Coma*   **FIGURE 1.24** *Marginal astigmatism*

4. Marginal Astigmatism (Also Known as Radial or Oblique Astigmatism)

Marginal astigmatism results when a small bundle of light strikes a lens from an oblique angle forming two line images of a point source (Figure 1.24). As a consequence, objects viewed obliquely through an ophthalmic lens may be blurred. Marginal astigmatism is often a source of discomfort to the patient and its reduction is an objective of corrected-curve lenses. However, all large lenses (over 52mm horizontal box measurement) exhibit peripheral distortion that cannot be eliminated.

5. Curvature of Field (Also Called Curvature of the Image)

Lenses do not form images of objects in a flat plane at the focal distance. Instead, curved images are formed concave toward the lenses (Figure 1.25). This aberration results from each object point being a different distance from the refracting surface. Reduction or elimination of curvature of field is another goal of corrected-curve lenses.

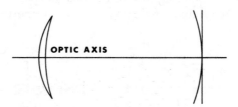

OPTIC AXIS

FIGURE 1.25 *Curvature of field*

6. Distortion

Distortion results from unequal magnification of object points not on the optical axis of a lens (Figure 1.26). When a patient looks through the periphery of a lens, the image is not in true proportion to the object. Through plus lenses, the image of a square has a pincushion appearance because the corners appear farther from the center than expected. When minus lenses are involved, the square appears barrel-shaped because the corners of the image seem closer to the center. Although lens curvatures designed to eliminate marginal astigmatism also reduce distortion, it is still necessary for patients to adjust to some effects of this aberration. There is apparent motion of objects when the head is turned, particularly with high power prescriptions. In addition, straight lines may appear curved, and curved objects distorted.

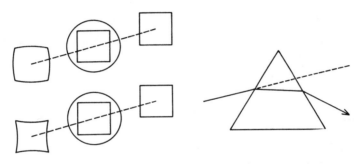

FIGURE 1.26 *Distortion*   **FIGURE 1.27** *Prism*

PRISM PRESCRIPTIONS

Prism prescriptions can be written independently or incorporated into a spherical, cylindrical, or sphero-cylinder correction. A prism lens does not converge or diverge light but instead deviates the rays passing through it. In certain cases, binocular vision cannot be achieved without this type of correction; in others, the patient is more comfortable when prisms are worn.

A prism is constructed with an apex (a thin edge) and a base (Figure 1.27). Light is deviated toward the base with the image projected in the direction of the apex. The unit of measurement is the prism diopter, indicated by the exponent[Δ]. One prism diopter deviates light 1cm at a distance of 1m on a tangent scale. This unit was suggested by Prentice (about 1890) because of its simplicity in computing and recording prism power.

PRISM EFFECTS IN A LENS

A prismatic effect is created when the patient looks away from the optical center of any plus or minus lens (Figures 1.28 and 1.29). This is easily visualized by noting that a convex lens may be considered a group of prisms with the bases touching at the center; conversely, a minus lens has its apexes coinciding at the center.

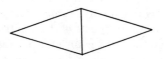

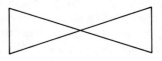

FIGURE 1.28 *Plus lens*   **FIGURE 1.29** *Minus lens*

If the patient looks away from the lens center, the effect is that of a prism with its base in, out, up, or down, depending upon the direction of the gaze and the power of the lens. Prismatic effect can be computed by applying Prentice's Law:

$$\text{prismatic effect} = \text{lens power} \times \text{decentration (in cm)}$$

Decentration is the distance from the center of the lens to the point in question. This distance is normally measured in millimeters and therefore must be converted to centimeters before applying the above formula.

PROBLEM:

Given a +5.00D lens, find the prismatic effect when the patient looks 15mm nasal to the optical center.

SOLUTION:

$$\begin{aligned}
\text{prismatic effect} &= F \times \text{decentration} \\
&= +5.00 \times 1\tfrac{1}{2} \text{ cm} \\
&= 7\tfrac{1}{2}^{\Delta} \text{ base out}
\end{aligned}$$

PROBLEM:

Given a −8.00D lens, find the prismatic effect when the patient looks 12mm below the optical center.

SOLUTION:

$$\begin{aligned}
\text{prismatic effect} &= F \times \text{decentration} \\
&= -8.00 \times 1.2\text{cm} \\
&= 9.6^\Delta \text{ base down} \\
&= 9\tfrac{3}{5}^\Delta \text{ base down}
\end{aligned}$$

When prism is to be incorporated into a prescription, sometimes it may be ordered by indicating the amount and direction of decentration. This is feasible only if the lens power is high enough and the lens blank of adequate size. When in doubt, query the laboratory.

PRISMATIC EFFECT WHEN TWO PRISMS ARE COMBINED

It is possible that the practitioner may want to know the combined effect of two prisms. This is determined by graphing the involved prismatic powers as illustrated in the following problems.

PROBLEM:

What is the resultant effect when the following prisms are combined?

2^Δ base up at $20°$

5^Δ base up at $70°$

PROCEDURE:

1. The prismatic powers are graphed along an "A" line and a "B" line. The "A" prism is the one whose position is closest to the numerical value zero.

   "A" prism $= 2^\Delta$ base up
   "B" prism $= 5^\Delta$ base up

2. "A" prism is plotted on the base line. "B" prism is constructed α degrees away. α is the difference between the two axes.

   $$70° - 20° = 50°$$

3. Graph prism "A" and prism "B" separated by α (50°). Complete the parallelogram (Figure 1.30). Draw the dotted line "R" from the point of origin to the opposite extremity of the parallelogram.

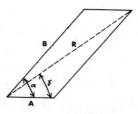

FIGURE 1.30

4. The dotted line "R" represents the prismatic effect. Measured "R" = 6½^Δ.

5. The base positioning is determined by adding the position of "A" to γ. γ is the angle between "A" and "R." γ = 36½°. The base positioning is 56½° (20° + 36½°).

SOLUTION:

Resultant prism = 6½^Δ base up at 56½°.

PROBLEM:

What is the resultant effect when the following prisms are combined?

6^Δ base down at 10°
5^Δ base down at 25°

PROCEDURE:

1. "A" prism is 6^Δ (positioned closest to numerical value zero). "B" prism is 5^Δ.

2. α = 25° − 10° = 15°

3. Graph prism "A" and prism "B" separated by α (15°) (Figure 1.31).

4. Measured "R" = 11^Δ

5. γ = 7° (angle between "A" and "R") γ, added to the positioning of "A" prism, = 17° (10° + 7°).

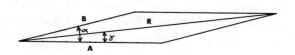

FIGURE 1.31

SOLUTION:

Resultant prism = 11^Δ base down at $17°$.

MEASUREMENT OF LENS AND/OR PRISM POWER

It is often necessary for the practitioner to determine the power of a lens prescription and/or if a prism correction has been incorporated. For example, if glasses have been worn, the dioptric and/or prism power needs to be ascertained before a new prescription is written. In addition, all prescriptions ordered from the laboratory must be checked for accuracy before dispensing to the patient.

It is customary to determine a lens prescription and/or the amount of prism incorporated by the use of a lensometer or vertexometer. The optical system of these instruments is such that it is possible to read the prescription directly from the dials after focusing the target. Each instrument has the manufacturer's instructions for its use.

There are two other methods of determining lens prescriptions, although rarely is either used for this purpose. One is hand neutralization and the other is the use of the lens gauge.

Instructions for Hand Neutralization

If the lens power is outside the limits of the lensometer, hand neutralization may be employed. Hand neutralization involves using a lens of known power to neutralize the motion seen through the lens of unknown power. It will be remembered that characteristically a lens of zero power demonstrates no motion, a spherical lens of plus power exhibits "against motion," and a minus spherical lens displays "with motion." A spherocylinder has different powers in the two principal meridians; therefore, the observed motion is neutralized by two different lenses corresponding to these meridians.

The lens to be neutralized must first be checked to see whether it is a sphere, cylinder, or sphero-cylinder. The observer holds the lens at arm's length and views a line object, such as the straight edge of a door or window. If the rotation produces a break in the continuity of the line, the lens is a cylinder or a sphero-cylinder; if there is no break, the lens is spherical. If an "against motion" is noted, the unknown lens is of plus power, and a minus lens is arbitrarily selected from the trial lens case for neutralization. By trial and error this process is repeated until both lenses placed together produce no motion. If the unknown lens shows a "with motion," the lens is minus power and plus lenses are selected for neutralization. In hand neutralizing sphero-cylinders, the two principal meridians are neutralized independently and the powers recorded on the optical cross. The prescription is then recorded as crossed cylinders and transposed into plus or minus cylinder form.

Note: The power of spherical, high plus lenses can also be found by holding the lens in front of an object and determining the best focus. Because the distance from the object to the lens is the focal length, its power is easily calculated.

Determining Lens Power with the Lens Gauge

Lens power can be ascertained by use of the lens gauge (sometimes referred to as a lens clock). This hand-held gauge, about 2 inches in diameter, is circular and has two outer fixed prongs with a movable pin between them. On the face of the clock are two concentric circles having numbers that indicate dioptric values. The black values of the inner circle denote the power of the convex surface of the lens; the red numbers of the outer circle give the power of the concave surface. In determining the lens power, the prongs of the clock are placed perpendicular on the lens surface.

If the hand does not move when the clock is rotated on either surface, the lens is spherical. The readings of both surfaces are added algebraically to give the approximate power of the lens (thickness is not taken into consideration).

If the hand on the face of the clock moves, the surface is cylindrical, the amount of cylinder being the difference between the highest and lowest readings. For example, if the hand moves from 7.00D to 9.00D and with further rotation back toward 7.00D, the cylinder is 2.00D. If this movement is observed on the convex surface, a plus cylinder is involved; if on the concave surface, a minus cylinder is involved. Because the axis and the meridian of maximum power are 90° apart, the clock must be turned through an angle of 90° to determine the maximal and minimal readings. To determine the prescription, the powers in the two principal meridians are each algebraically combined with the spherical power of the opposite surface.

For example, the clock reading for the concave lens surface is −7.00D. The convex surface reads +7.00D in the 90° meridian and +8.00D in the 180°. Therefore, the prescription is Plano + 1.00 × 90°.

From a practical viewpoint, lens clocks are used only to determine the curvature of a particular surface and/or to ascertain the cylinder design. The practitioner usually checks the curves of the lenses the patient is wearing. If he wishes to prescribe the same lens form or use other specific lens designs, the lens clock is utilized to confirm laboratory accuracy. It is also used to check bitoric effects (cylinder on both surfaces) of plastic lenses after they are mounted (see Chapter 7, "Plastic Ophthalmic Lenses").

Lens gauges are calibrated for an index of 1.53. If the lens is manufactured of plastic or of glass having another index, determination of approximate power needs to be made. The conversion formula is as follows:

$$F = R\left(\frac{n - 1}{c - 1}\right)$$

F = true power of the lens
R = reading on the lens gauge
n = index of the lens
c = index for which the clock is calibrated

PROBLEM:

The total power of a lens as determined with a lens gauge is +6.00D. Find the true power if the index of the lens is 1.60.

SOLUTION:

$$F_{true} = R\left(\frac{n - 1}{c - 1}\right)$$

$$= +6.00D\left(\frac{1.60 - 1}{1.53 - 1}\right)$$

$$= +6.80D$$

PROBLEM:

The total power of a lens as determined with a lens gauge is −4.50D. Find the true power if the index of the lens is 1.47.

SOLUTION:

$$F_{true} = R\left(\frac{n - 1}{c - 1}\right)$$

$$= -4.50\left(\frac{1.47 - 1}{1.53 - 1}\right)$$

$$= -3.96D$$

PROBLEM:

If the true power of a lens of index 1.50 is +5.00D, what is the lens gauge reading?

SOLUTION:

$$F_{true} = R \left(\frac{n-1}{c-1} \right)$$

$$+5.00 = R \left(\frac{1.50-1}{1.53-1} \right)$$

$$R = +5.30D$$

PROBLEM:

If a $-4.00D$ lens has a lens gauge reading of $-4.25D$, what is the index of the lens?

SOLUTION:

$$F_{true} = R \left(\frac{n-1}{c-1} \right)$$

$$-4.00 = -4.25 \left(\frac{n-1}{1.53-1} \right)$$

$$(n-1) = 0.47$$

$$n = 1.47$$

Chapter 2

INTRODUCTION TO BIFOCAL LENSES

HISTORY OF BIFOCAL LENSES

A bifocal lens is an ingenious device having two focal lengths in one lens. It is used primarily for the correction of presbyopia (the technical term for the diminishing plasticity of the crystalline lens). This condition necessitates additional plus power at near and usually becomes critical in the midforties. Bifocals are also used in cases of muscle imbalance where the patient needs more plus at near for comfortable vision.

Benjamin Franklin invented the bifocal lens to eliminate the inconvenience of using separate pairs of glasses for distance and near. The solution seems so logical, it is surprising that this lens form did not appear until 1784. The original Franklin bifocal featured a halved distance lens and a halved near correction placed in juxtaposition and held together by a circular metal-rimmed frame. The principle behind this split bifocal is seen in the modern straight-across design.

It was inevitable that the convenience and practical value of a multifocal lens design would result in improved versions. The first one-piece bifocal (change in power for near achieved through a change in curvature of one surface) appeared to have its beginning in 1837. Called the Solid Upcurve Bifocal, it was patented by Isaac Schnaitman of Philadelphia and was manufactured so that the top portion of a biconvex lens was ground flat on one surface. The finished lens was, therefore, a combination of a plano-convex and a biconvex lens.

Two more bifocal designs were patented in 1888 by August Marich. One, known as the Perfection Bifocal, had the same basic principle as the Benjamin Franklin split bifocal. Two separate pieces of crown glass were utilized, with the segment area being semicircular in appearance. The other bifocal featured a crown glass major lens to which was cemented a "wafer" of spherical power equivalent to the near add. It was known as the Cement Bifocal. Canada balsam, the adhesive used, presented many problems. Under warm conditions the segment tended to slide; in cold weather the wafer would sometimes break away from the major lens. In addition, regardless of how skilled the optician was in cementing the segment, aberrations were present that interfered with clarity of vision. Later another cement lens, known as Opifex Bifocal, was introduced. It somewhat improved upon the original design, but the obvious disadvantages of using cement to attach the plus power wafer were still present.

The first attempt at gaining additional power at near by using a glass button of a higher index of refraction was made by John Borsch, Sr., in 1899. A countersink curve was formed on the convex surface of the major blank into which was cemented a small flint segment. In the final step of manufacture a cover lens of crown glass was cemented over the entire front surface of the lens. This bifocal design was called the Kryptok lens, named after the Greek word *kryptos* meaning "hidden."

In 1908 John Borsch, Jr., invented the first fused bifocal, retaining the name of his father's original lens design, Kryptok. A round segment button was fused into a major blank that had been prepared by removing a section into which the higher index segment could be fused. The near power was controlled by the ratio of the two indices and the radius of the countersink curve.

The first one-piece bifocals to be available widely were manufactured in 1910 by Continental Optical Co. The lens series was distributed under the trade name Ultex and is still produced today.

In 1926 the bifocal that has been the most popular to date was introduced by Univis Lens Co. Of fused construction, it featured a straight dividing line, which eliminated the superfluous upper area of the round segment. This resulted in an optical center located closer to the top of the segment, thereby reducing the amount of image jump. Since its introduction, it has been copied with minor modifications by every major lens manufacturer.

The next bifocal that proved extremely successful was a one-piece, straight-across design similar in appearance to the original Benjamin

Franklin split bifocal. Introduced by American Optical Corp. in the later 1950s, it is distributed under the trade name Executive.

Although bifocal lenses enabled a presbyope the convenience of clear, near vision without changing glasses, some patients objected to the appearance of the dividing line, feeling it was a telltale sign of maturity. As a result, lens manufacturers attempted to produce a bifocal without a dividing line. The first relatively successful effort was the Younger Seamless bifocal designed in the middle 1950s. The sharp line of demarcation of conventional bifocals was polished out. However, it had its drawbacks in that this blending resulted in a blurred area with an uncontrollable cylindrical power at an oblique axis.

MODERN BIFOCAL DESIGNS

There are two basic forms of construction used in the manufacture of contemporary bifocals. The fused bifocal features a crown glass major lens blank, usually of 1.523 index, for the distance correction. The near prescription is obtained by fusing a segment of higher index into a designated countersink curve in the major blank. Most quality bifocal manufacturers prefer barium segments whenever possible because the low dispersion factor and relative hardness make this a practical type of segment glass. However, flint glass is sometimes combined with barium to give the higher index of refraction necessary for certain segment powers.

The other basic bifocal design features a "one-piece" form of construction. The change in near power results from a change in curvature on one surface of the lens. All bifocals utilizing a high-index glass for a distance correction and all bifocals made of plastic are of a one-piece construction. Some one-piece designs are available in crown glass.

One-piece bifocals, with the exception of the seamless (blended) design, can be identified by a ridge that divides the distance correction from the near. It is felt by moving a finger across the segment side of the lens. Because a fused bifocal has a button designed to fit the countersink curve and the spherical curve of the segment is the same as the distance correction, a ridge is not present.

TYPES OF BIFOCAL DESIGNS

Fused and one-piece bifocal lenses of contemporary design are further subdivided into five basic types. The classifications are determined by the shape of the segment.

1.   Round-top bifocals
2.   Straight-top bifocals
3.   Curved-top bifocals
4.   Straight-across bifocals
5.   "Invisible" bifocals

1. Round-top Bifocals

The round-top bifocal is constructed in such a manner that the segment forms a perfect circle. However, when the lenses are cut to fit the frame, the segments are almost always semicircular in shape. Round-top bifocals are produced in both fused and one-piece designs. By the nature of their construction the optical center of the segment is the exact center of the original round button.

2. Straight-top Bifocals (Also Known as Flat-top Bifocals)

Lenses that fall into this category feature a straight line division that does not extend to either the nasal or temporal extremity in the factory blank. However, when the bifocal lens is cut and edged to fit a specific frame, it is possible, although unusual, that the segment line may reach one or both edges of the lens. These lenses may be fused or one-piece in construction.

The majority of straight-top bifocals feature segments with upper corners that are sharply outlined; some are manufactured with the upper limits rounded in shape. The most often prescribed are designed in such a manner that the lower edge of the segment forms a semicircular pattern. A limited few feature straight lines for both upper and lower extremities.

Almost since its introduction, the straight-top bifocal has been the most popular of the modern multifocal designs. The relatively useless upper area of the round-top segment is eliminated, allowing the patient to hold his head in a more normal position when using the widest area of the segment.

3. Curved-top Bifocals

This category consists of bifocals featuring a curved dividing line with the lower segment edge always circular in shape. The outer limits of the dividing line are either sharp or rounded, depending on the particular design.

4. Straight-across Bifocals

This bifocal design is always a one-piece construction. The dividing line is an inverted "shelf" extending from the nasal to the temporal edges of the nonocular surface of the lens. This multifocal design is a sophisticated version of the original Benjamin Franklin split bifocal. Both feature the "no jump" principle since the optical centers of the distance and near prescriptions are at the dividing line.

5. "Invisible" Bifocal Designs

The seamless (blended) are the bifocal designs in this category. They are discussed in Chapter 5, "Prescribing 'Invisible' Multifocals."

MATHEMATICAL COMPUTATIONS INVOLVING FUSED BIFOCALS

To understand bifocal design better, some of the mathematical calculations involved in determining the specifications for proper adds in bifocal corrections are given.

The dioptric power of the add of a fused bifocal is determined by the relationship of the index of the glass used in the distance correction and the higher index of the glass used in the near portion. These indices, in turn, determine the power of the countersink curve needed to give the additional dioptric power in the segment (Figure 2.1).

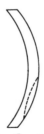

FIGURE 2.1 *Countersink curve*

The formulas used in these calculations are as follows:

$$F_i = \frac{n_n - 1}{n_d - 1} \times F_{front}$$

F_i = power change caused by the change in indices
n_n = index of the near add
n_d = index of the distance correction
F_{front} = dioptric curvature of the front surface

$$F_{gain} = F_i - F_{front}$$

F_{gain} = power gained by the change in indices
F_i = power change caused by the change in indices
F_{front} = dioptric curvature of the front surface

$$F_{needed} = F_{add} - F_{gain}$$

F_{needed} = additional power to give total power of the segment
F_{add} = total add power
F_{gain} = power gained by the change in indices

$$r = \frac{n_d - n_n}{F_{needed}}$$

r = radius of the countersink curve in meters
n_d = index of the distance correction
n_n = index of the near add
F_{needed} = additional power needed to give total power of the segment

$$F_{cc} = \frac{n_d - 1}{r}$$

F_{cc} = dioptric power of the countersink curve
n_d = index of the distance correction
r = radius of the countersink curve

$$F_{rf} = F_{ocular} + F_{cc}$$

F_{rf} = dioptric power of reading field
F_{ocular} = dioptric power of ocular surface of the lens
F_{cc} = dioptric power of countersink curve

PROBLEM:

A round-top fused bifocal has a distance power of +6.00D; the add is +3.00D. The inside of the lens is −8.00D. The distance index is 1.523; the near index is 1.62. Find the following:
(a) the radius of the countersink curve
(b) the power of the countersink curve
(c) the power of the reading field before fusing

PROCEDURE FOR (a):

1. Determine the power change caused by the change in indices.

$$F_i = \frac{n_n - 1}{n_d - 1} \times F_{front}$$

$$= \frac{1.62 - 1}{1.523 - 1} \times 14$$

$$= 16.6D$$

2.   Determine the power gained because of the index.

$$\mathbf{F}_{gain} = \mathbf{F}_i - \mathbf{F}_{front}$$
$$= 16.6 - 14.0$$
$$= 2.6D$$

3.   Determine the power needed.

$$\mathbf{F}_{needed} = \mathbf{F}_{add} - \mathbf{F}_{gain}$$
$$= 3.00 - 2.60$$
$$= 0.40D$$

4.   Determine the radius of the countersink curve.

$$r = \frac{n_d - n_n}{F_{needed}}$$
$$= \frac{1.523 - 1.62}{0.40}$$
$$= -0.24m$$

SOLUTION TO (a):

Countersink curve radius $= -0.24m$

PROCEDURE FOR (b):

Determine the power of the countersink curve.

$$\mathbf{F}_{cc} = \frac{n_d - 1}{r}$$
$$= \frac{1.523 - 1}{-0.24}$$
$$= -2.18D$$

SOLUTION TO (b):

Countersink curve power $= -2.18D$

PROCEDURE FOR (c):

Determine the power of the reading field before fusing.

$$F_{rf} = F_{ocular} + F_{cc}$$
$$= -8.00 + (-2.18)$$
$$= -10.18D$$

Solution to (c):

Power of the reading field before fusing $= -10.18D$

Problem:

A round-top fused bifocal has a distance power of $-4.00D$; the add is $+2.00D$. The inside curve of the lens is $-10.00D$. The near index is 1.60. Find the following:
(a) the radius of the countersink curve
(b) the power of the countersink curve
(c) the power of the reading field before fusing
(d) the thickness of the button
Assume the distance index is 1.523 and the segment is a 22mm round.

Procedure for (a):

1.   Determine the power change caused by the index.

$$F_i = \frac{n_n - 1}{n_d - 1} \times F_{front}$$

$$= \frac{1.60 - 1}{1.523 - 1} \times 6$$

$$= 6.90D$$

2.   Determine the power gained because of the index.

$$F_{gain} = F_i - F_{front}$$
$$= 6.9 - 6.0$$
$$= 0.9D$$

3.   Determine the power needed.

$$F_{needed} = F_{add} - F_{gain}$$
$$= +2.00 - 0.9$$
$$= +1.10D$$

4.   Determine the radius of the countersink curve.

$$r = \frac{n_d - n_n}{F_{needed}}$$

$$= \frac{1.523 - 1.6}{1.10}$$

$$= -0.07\text{m}$$

SOLUTION TO (a):

Countersink curve radius $= -0.07$m

PROCEDURE FOR (b):

Determine the power of the countersink curve.

$$F_{cc} = \frac{n_d - 1}{r}$$

$$= \frac{1.523 - 1}{-0.07}$$

$$= -7.50\text{D}$$

SOLUTION TO (b):

Power of the countersink curve $= -7.50$D

PROCEDURE FOR (c):

Determine the power of the reading field before fusing.

$$F_{rf} = F_{ocular} + F_{cc}$$
$$= -10.00 + (-7.5)$$
$$= -17.50\text{D}$$

SOLUTION TO (c):

Power of the reading field before fusing $= -17.50$D

PROCEDURE FOR (d):

Determine the thickness of the button using the sagittal (thickness) formula.

$$\text{Sag} = \frac{(F_{front} - F_{cc})(\text{½ seg diameter})^2}{2(n_d - 1)}$$

$$= \frac{13.5(.011)^2}{2(1.523 - 1)}$$

$$= .0016\text{m} = 1.6\text{mm}$$

Solution to (d):

Thickness of the button = 1.6mm

Problem:

A 22mm round-segment bifocal has a distance prescription of +4.00 −1.00 × 45, add +3.50D. The index of the distance portion is 1.523, and the index of the segment is 1.6. The inside curve of the lens is −5.00D. Find the following:
(a) the radius of the countersink curve
(b) the power of the countersink curve
(c) the power of the reading field before fusing
(d) the Kryptok factor (factory term for dioptric change in countersink curve that increases add by 1 diopter)
(e) the thickness of the button

Procedure for (a):

1. Determine the power change caused by the change in indices.

    Note: Since fused bifocals are manufactured in minus cylinder form, the cylinder is on the back surface and not taken into consideration when determining F_{front} curvature. If the prescription is written in plus cylinder form, transpose to minus using the new written correction to determine F_{front} (outside curvature).

    $$F_i = \frac{n_n - 1}{n_d - 1} \times F_{front}$$
    $$= \frac{1.60 - 1}{1.523 - 1} \times 9$$
    $$= +10.33D$$

2. Determine the power gained because of the index.

    $$F_{gain} = F_i - F_{front}$$
    $$= +10.33 - 9.00$$
    $$= +1.33D$$

3. Determine the power needed.

    $$F_{needed} = F_{add} - F_{gain}$$
    $$= +3.50 - (+1.33)$$
    $$= +2.17D$$

4. Determine the radius of the countersink curve.

$$r = \frac{n_d - n_n}{F_{needed}}$$
$$= \frac{1.523 - 1.6}{+2.17}$$
$$= -0.0355 \text{m}$$

SOLUTION TO (a):

Countersink curve radius $= -0.0355$m

PROCEDURE FOR (b):

Determine the power of the countersink curve.

$$F_{cc} = \frac{n_d - 1}{r}$$
$$= \frac{1.523 - 1}{-0.0355}$$
$$= -14.73 \text{D}$$

SOLUTION TO (b):

Countersink curve power $= -14.73$D

PROCEDURE FOR (c):

Determine the power of the reading field before fusing.

$$F_{rf} = F_{ocular} + F_{cc}$$
$$= -5.00 + (-14.73)$$
$$= -19.73 \text{D}$$

SOLUTION TO (c):

Power of the reading field before fusing $= -19.73$D

PROCEDURE FOR (d):

Determine the Kryptok factor.

$$K_f = \frac{n_d - 1}{n_n - n_d}$$
$$= \frac{1.523 - 1.00}{1.60 - 1.523}$$
$$= 6.79$$

SOLUTION TO (d):

Kryptok factor = 6.79

PROCEDURE FOR (e):

Determine the thickness of the segment button.

$$t = \frac{(F_{front} - F_{cc})h^2}{2(n_d - 1)}$$
$$= \frac{[+9.00 - (-14.73)](0.011)^2}{2(1.523 - 1)}$$
$$= 0.00275m = 2.75mm$$

SOLUTION TO (e):

Segment button thickness = 2.75mm

PROBLEM:

A round-top 24mm bifocal has a distance power of $-5.00 - 1.50 \times 10$. The add is +3.00D. The inside curve of the lens is -8.00D. The index of the distance portion of the lens is 1.5, and the index of the segment is 1.6. Find the following:
(a) the radius of the countersink curve
(b) the power of the countersink curve
(c) the power of the reading field before fusing
(d) the Kryptok factor (the term remains by common usage)
(e) the thickness of the button

PROCEDURE FOR (a):

1. Determine the power change caused by the change in indices.

$$F_i = \frac{n_n - 1}{n_d - 1} \times F_{front}$$
$$= \frac{1.6 - 1}{1.5 - 1} \times 3$$
$$= 3.6D$$

2. Determine the power gained because of the index.

$$F_{gain} = F_i - F_{front}$$
$$= 3.6 - 3.0$$
$$= 0.60D$$

3.   Determine the power needed.

$$F_{needed} = F_{add} - F_{gain}$$
$$= 3.0 - 0.60$$
$$= 2.40D$$

4.   Determine the radius of the countersink curve.

$$r = \frac{n_d - n_n}{F_{needed}}$$
$$= \frac{1.5 - 1.6}{2.4}$$
$$= -0.0417m$$

SOLUTION TO (a):

Countersink curve radius $= -0.0417m$.

PROCEDURE FOR (b):

Determine the power of the countersink curve.

$$F_{cc} = \frac{n_d - 1}{r}$$
$$= \frac{1.5 - 1}{-0.0417}$$
$$= -12.00D$$

SOLUTION TO (b):

Countersink curve power $= -12.00D$

PROCEDURE FOR (c):

Determine the power of the reading field before fusing.

$$F_{rf} = F_{ocular} + F_{cc}$$
$$= -8.00 + (-12.00)$$
$$= -20.00D$$

SOLUTION TO (c):

Reading field power before fusing $= -20.00D$

PROCEDURE FOR (d):

Determine the Kryptok factor.

$$K_f = \frac{n_d - 1}{n_n - n_d}$$
$$= \frac{1.5 - 1}{1.6 - 1.5}$$
$$= 5$$

SOLUTION TO (d):

Kryptok factor = 5

PROCEDURE FOR (e):

Determine the thickness of the segment button.

$$t = \frac{(F_{front} - F_{cc})h^2}{2(n_d - 1)}$$
$$= \frac{[3.00 - (-12.00)](0.012)^2}{2(1.5 - 1)}$$
$$= 0.0022m = 2.2mm$$

SOLUTION TO (e):

Segment button thickness = 2.2mm

Chapter 3

PRESCRIBING MODERN GLASS BIFOCAL DESIGNS

INTRODUCTION

Contemporary bifocal lenses intended for general-purpose wear or prescribed for vocational/avocational purposes are available to fill the needs of every patient requiring such a correction. The popular designs are manufactured from both glass and plastic. This chapter concerns itself with conventional glass bifocals. Chapter 7, "Plastic Ophthalmic Lenses," analyzes the hard resin (CR39) plastic designs and polycarbonate lenses.

Lenses are illustrated with explanations of prescribing considerations; trade names are used when the particular design is identified with its creator and/or its distributor.

Note: Bifocals manufactured in special forms, such as photochromic and cataract lenses, are covered in the chapters involving those areas: Chapter 9, "Prescribing Absorptive Lenses," and Chapter 11, "Lenses for Special Uses."

Glass bifocals can have either a fused or one-piece construction. (All plastic bifocals are one-piece.) Fused-glass bifocals manufactured in the

United States are in minus cylinder form with the segment fused on the outside surface. The major blank is fashioned of crown glass, index 1.523; the segment is of a higher index, either barium or a combination of barium-flint. A very few are made exclusively of flint glass. Flint results in more chromatic aberration, so most manufacturers limit its content, although the higher index of refraction makes it a necessity for certain high-add lenses.

One-piece glass bifocals are either plus or minus cylinder form although manufacturers in the United States are discontinuing the plus cylinder design. All are fashioned of crown glass, index 1.523, except for a few constructed of high-index glass. These are intended for strong minus corrections and are identified in the text. When a finger is run over the segment side of a one-piece bifocal, the ridge dividing the distance from the near area can be felt. This method is frequently used to distinguish fused bifocals from the one-piece designs.

Theoretically, one-piece bifocals fashioned of crown glass have less chromatic aberration and are lighter than the fused designs, which by necessity utilize the heavier barium and/or flint segments. Practically speaking, however, patients notice little difference, except of course in cases of high-index glass lenses. Therefore, the design recommended to the patient depends on its optical characteristics: position of segment optical center, width of segment, etc.

IMAGE JUMP VS. OBJECT DISPLACEMENT

At one time it was felt that a patient needing a bifocal with a plus distance correction should be prescribed a round-top design because the low placement of the segment optical center reduces or eliminates the base-up effect of the distance when viewing near objects. (Base-up was neutralized by the base-down because the patient looked above the segment optical center when reading.) Today, practitioners feel the reduction of image jump as the patient's eye travels from distance to near is more critical. Since image jump is controlled by the segment optical center (the closer the optical center is to the division, the less the image jump), contemporary bifocals of a straight-top design with an optical center 3 to 5mm below the dividing line are preferred for most prescriptions. (Lenses that have a segment optical center at the dividing line lack cosmetic appeal.) These bifocals allow the patient to hold the neck and head in relatively normal positions, thus allowing for comfortable near viewing; the widest part of the segment (through the optical center) is reached almost as soon as the line of sight passes into the add power.

STRAIGHT-TOP FUSED BIFOCAL SEGMENTS WITH SHARP CORNERS AND ROUNDED LOWER EXTREMITIES

These fused lenses produced by all major manufacturers are the most widely prescribed glass bifocals in the United States. The impractical upper area of a round segment button is eliminated, resulting in a segment optical center ranging from 3 to 5mm below the dividing line (depending on the design), thus minimizing image jump.

There are several recent changes involving the manufacturers of these lenses. Univis, Inc., who developed the design under the name Univis D, sold its lens division to Vision-Ease in 1982/83. This company retained only the "D" to identify the straight-top/flat-top series. Bausch & Lomb, Inc., who released the designs under the trade name Orthogon straight-top, no longer manufactures multifocals. The lenses are currently distributed by major manufacturers under the following trade names:

MANUFACTURER	TRADE NAME
Vision-Ease	D series
American Optical Corp.	Tillyer S
Shuron-Textron (formerly Shuron-Continental)	Kurova D
Titmus Optical Co.	Flat-top series

Straight-top 22 (22mm × 16mm)

At one time, this was a widely prescribed bifocal. However, most manufacturers are phasing out the size as the ST25mm and ST28mm are considered general-purpose bifocals that better fill the need for an adequate near field. The ST22mm has a segment optical center 5mm below the dividing line, except for the Vision-Ease version, which is made with an optical center 4mm below (Figure 3.1). The original ST18mm, 19mm, and 20mm lenses have not been available for decades.

Straight-top 25 (25mm × 17mm)

This bifocal was originally intended as a compromise general-purpose and occupational lens for patients requiring a relatively large segment. The use of larger frames and the increase in occupations involving a great deal of close work have emphasized the importance of the ST25mm. The most prescribed size in the United States, it is usually recommended for the first-time wearer and used to replace the ST22mm when the

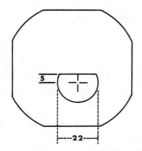

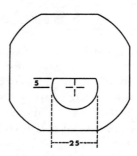

FIGURE 3.1   *Straight-top 22*   **FIGURE 3.2**   *Straight-top 25*

patient needs a new bifocal correction. The segment optical center is 5mm below the dividing line, except for the Vision-Ease design, which is 4mm below (Figure 3.2).

Straight-top 28 (28mm × 19mm)

The ST28mm was designed as an occupational lens for patients requiring a large segment area. It was recommended only for accountants, teachers, secretaries, and others involved in many hours of near work. Today, in view of the comfort it affords, practitioners often prescribe it as a general-purpose bifocal. Because the optical center is 5mm below the dividing line, the ST28mm can provide horizontal prism at the near point when such a need is indicated (Figure 3.3). Although overdecentration results in a less usable near area, this method of obtaining prism at the reading level is superior both optically and cosmetically to a factory-ground prism segment.

Straight-top 35 (35mm × 22.5mm)

The ST35 is usually limited to patients requiring an occupational bifocal. Like all large-segment lenses, its cosmetic appearance is not as pleasing as bifocals that utilize a smaller reading area. The dividing line becomes especially prominent when a high add is involved. Most manufacturers place the optical center 3mm below the dividing line (Figure 3.4). Titmus places it at the segment line and calls the lens Thinlite Ultrasite. Vision-Ease sets it 5mm below.

Note: The ST45, a fused bifocal having a horizontal measurement of 45mm, has been discontinued. Thus, the ST35 is the widest available glass lens in this basic style.

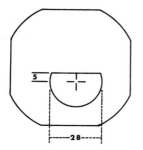

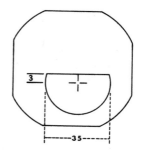

FIGURE 3.3 *Straight-top 28*   **FIGURE 3.4** *Straight-top 35*

UNIQUE STRAIGHT-TOP FUSED DESIGNS

Univis I.S. (Identifiable Segment) (22mm × 16mm)

The Identifiable Segment, a 22mm flat-top glass bifocal with curved corners and rounded lower extremities is no longer available. It was prescribed as a general-wear bifocal, but the size and appearance limited its use (Figure 3.5).

Note: A similar-looking lens was Shuron-Continental's Ultex K, one of the original straight-top designs. This discontinued one-piece bifocal in plus cylinder form was made in two sizes, 19mm × 14mm and 22.5mm × 16.5mm.

B-Style (26mm × 9mm and 22mm × 9mm)

The B is a rarely prescribed lens. Because of its long, narrow appearance, it is sometimes referred to as the "ribbon" or "bar" segment. Although its horizontal size varies, the vertical remains a constant 9mm. The optical center is 4.5mm below the segment line, with the upper and lower divisions straight lines of equal length (Figure 3.6). Its purpose is to

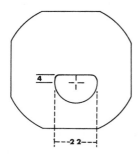

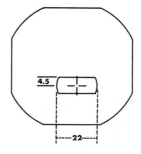

FIGURE 3.5 *Univis I.S.*   **FIGURE 3.6** *B segment*

give an injury-prone patient distant vision beneath the near area. To accomplish this, the segment needs to be set at least 17mm high. These bifocals should be prescribed in conjunction with single-vision reading glasses. They are too small for prolonged pleasurable near viewing.

Note: The original B segment was available exclusively from Univis. When Vision-Ease took over the company, the 28mm × 9mm size was discontinued.

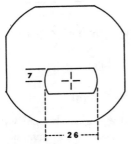

FIGURE 3.7   *R segment*   **FIGURE 3.8**   *Prism segment*

R-style (26mm × 14mm and 22mm × 14mm)

The upper and lower limits of the R segment are straight lines of equal length, with an optical center 7mm below the dividing line (Figure 3.7). Originated by Univis, the lens was rarely prescribed because the two division lines resulted in a prominent-looking bifocal; the positioning of the optical center creates more image jump than a straight-top D-style segment. Vision-Ease has discontinued the 28 × 14mm size.

Note: R-compensating bifocals (the standard R described above is #7 in the series) are available from Vision-Ease. However, their use is not a recommended method of compensating for vertical imbalance at the near point. They are discussed in Chapter 13, "Vertical Imbalance at the Reading Level."

PRISM SEGMENTS

The only prism segment manufactured today in the United States is distributed by Vision-Ease. The segment is a "ribbon-type" design with a vertical height of 10mm (Figure 3.8). It is available only with prism base-in. The amount of prism desired is ordered and a computer determines the horizontal width of the segment. It usually hovers about 22mm across.

Prism segment bifocals are so rare that most practitioners have never seen them. The reasons for not prescribing these lenses:

1. Cosmetic appearance: The segment looks like a miniature prism "tacked" onto a major lens and results in an unsightly, weird-looking design.
2. There is pronounced distortion through the segment as a result of the prism.
3. Color aberration: Patients see color fringes around reading material.
4. Near field of view is limited.

If a patient needs horizontal prism at near, it should be obtained by overdecentering a ST28mm or ST35mm bifocal having a segment optical center 5mm or 3mm below the dividing line. If the full prismatic amount cannot be obtained by this method, a separate pair of single-vision reading glasses with the total recommended correction can be prescribed for prolonged near work.

Note: Bausch & Lomb at one time made available Panoptik Prism Segments with prism base-down and base-up for use in correction of vertical imbalance. Such lenses are no longer manufactured.

CURVED-TOP FUSED BIFOCALS WITH SHARP CORNERS

This design was developed by American Optical Corp. and originally distributed under the trade name Ful-Vue bifocal (later changed to Tillyer C and then to Tillyer Sovereign). It has the same basic optical properties as the straight-top D-style bifocal, although the segment features a slightly curved dividing line. The optical center of all sizes available in the Tillyer Sovereign is 4.5mm below the dividing line. A comparable lens is available from Vision-Ease with an optical center 4mm or 5mm (noted in the explanation).

C-22 (22mm × 15mm)

The curved-top 22mm was designed as a general-purpose bifocal (Figure 3.9). The Vision-Ease version has an optical center 4mm below the dividing line. However, its small segment size makes it a rarely prescribed lens.

Note: The original series included a C-20 that is no longer available.

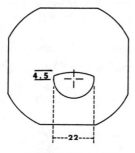
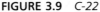

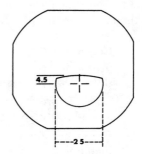

FIGURE 3.9   *C-22*   FIGURE 3.10   *Curved-top 25*

C-25 (25mm × 17mm)

This size, originally considered a compromise general-purpose/occupational bifocal, functions in the same manner as the ST25mm design (Figure 3.10). However, the latter is more widely used because it has an edge in cosmetic appeal. The Vision-Ease version has an optical center 4mm below the segment dividing line.

Vision-Ease C-28 (28mm × 18.5mm)

The basic design of the Tillyer Sovereign is available from Vision-Ease in a 28mm horizontal size with an optical center 5mm below the dividing line (Figure 3.11). Prescribed as a large-segment, general-purpose lens, it can be used like the ST28mm bifocal. However, the latter has a slightly less noticeable dividing line.

CURVED-TOP FUSED BIFOCALS WITH CURVED CORNERS

This design was originated by Bausch & Lomb under the trade name Orthogon Panoptik. It has a slightly curved dividing line with the upper segment extremities forming curved corners. The original Panoptik was available in two sizes: 22m × 14mm and 24mm × 16.5mm with the segment optical center 4.5mm below the dividing line. Bausch & Lomb has discontinued manufacture of all multifocals, but the basic design is available from Vision-Ease.

P-24 (Vision-Ease)

This lens is rarely prescribed. It serves the same purpose as the ST25mm, which has a slightly larger near area and a less noticeable segment. The segment optical center is 4mm below the dividing line (Figure 3.12).

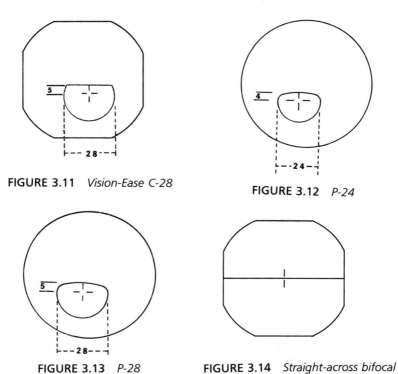

FIGURE 3.11 *Vision-Ease C-28*

FIGURE 3.12 *P-24*

FIGURE 3.13 *P-28*

FIGURE 3.14 *Straight-across bifocal*

P-28 (Vision-Ease)

The P-28 is a general-wear, large-segment bifocal that serves the same purpose as the ST28mm. It is rarely prescribed since the alternative is cosmetically more attractive. The segment optical center is 5mm below the dividing line (Figure 3.13).

THE STRAIGHT-ACROSS (EXECUTIVE) BIFOCAL

The straight-across, minus cylinder, one-piece design was created by American Optical Corp. under the trade name Executive bifocal (Figure 3.14). It is distributed by other manufacturers under the following trade names:

MANUFACTURER	TRADE NAME
Shuron-Textron	Kurova M
Titmus Optical Co.	Horizon
Vision-Ease	Bifield

This lens is considered an occupational bifocal. The segment extends from nasal to temporal extremities of the factory blank. Image jump is eliminated because the optical center is positioned at the dividing line. Laboratories are stressing that the Executive bifocal is not suitable for oversize frames. Although available in large blanks, the construction results in a relatively thick lens, making the glass version difficult to wear comfortably. The cosmetic disadvantage lies in the obvious inverted "shelves" located on the outside surface. These tend to chip, particularly when high add glass designs are involved. The ST35mm may prove more satisfactory as an occupational bifocal.

ROUND-TOP FUSED BIFOCALS

Round-top bifocals, so called because the segments are a completed circle in the original factory blank, almost always give the effect of a slightly full half-circle when cut to ordered segment height.

Some discontinued Bausch & Lomb trade names had become synonymous with round-top fused glass lenses: Orthogon C (16mm round), Orthogon D (20mm round), and Orthogon F (22mm round). American Optical called both the 20 and 22mm round by the same name, Tillyer D. Today, major manufacturers do not make a stock bifocal blank smaller than a 22mm round. However, fused round segments can be ground to a smaller diameter. For example, the round 16mm was originally intended as a golfer's bifocal set low in the finished lens so that the golfer could utilize the distance correction without interference. The size can still be ordered if desired.

Quality round-top 22mm bifocals are sometimes confused with the Kryptok lens available from numerous optical companies. The latter is designed to keep production costs at a minimum (manufacturers processing the Kryptok may not maintain the high standards required of quality lenses). In most cases, the type of glass used in the Kryptok segment causes high chromatic aberration that the patient sees as colored fringes around reading material.

Round-top 22 (22mm round segment)

The round-top 22mm lens is designed as a general-purpose bifocal (Figure 3.15). However, positioning of the optical center (11mm below the segment line) results in considerable image jump, as well as an uncomfortable head tilt when reaching the maximum near width. If the patient's primary concern is a cosmetic one, the segment is less visible than a comparably sized straight-top or curved-top design. (In the lower adds, especially, it is difficult to see). There are also patients who adapt more readily to and are more comfortable with the round-top bifocal because the change from distance to near is not exaggerated as with straight segment designs. The personality of the patient is the key factor in the recommendation of the round-top 22mm bifocal.

Note: Catalogues currently list 24, 25, and 35mm round-segment fused bifocals as available from various manufacturers, but they are rarely prescribed.

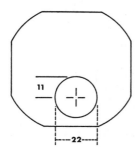

FIGURE 3.15 *Round-top 22*

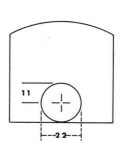

FIGURE 3.16 *Ultex B*

ROUND-TOP ONE-PIECE BIFOCALS

Ultex B (22mm Round)

Ultex B was the trade name for Shuron-Textron's 22mm round one-piece glass bifocal in plus cylinder form (Figure 3.16). The Orthogon B by Bausch & Lomb and the Tillyer B by American Optical were comparable lenses. This bifocal style used to be prescribed for the same cases as a 22mm round-top fused design, but plus cylinder lenses are no longer used in the United States.

Ultex E (32mm × 16mm)

The Ultex E is a plus cylinder lens, semicircular in shape and measuring 32mm across at its widest point, the lowest extremity of the lens (Figure 3.17). In the manufacturing process one large blank with a 32mm round segment is split through the center. The result is two lenses, each having an optical center 16mm down from the top of the dividing line (with considerable image jump). Designed as compromise general-purpose occupational lenses, Ultex E bifocals were phased out by manufacturers in the United States (the shape/size is still used for some high-add designs for the low-vision patient).

Ultex A (38mm × 19mm)

The Ultex A is a semicircular segment measuring 38mm across at its widest point, with an optical center 19mm below the dividing line (Figure 3.18). The manufacturing process is like that of the Ultex E. When the bevel allowance is made, the maximum segment height is 18mm or 18.5mm. If a higher segment is needed, the practitioner specifies Ultex AA (sometimes called Ultex AL; Figure 3.19). The manufacturer then utilizes one factory blank to obtain a single finished lens. Designed as a vocational bifocal, the style was unique at its conception, offering an exceptionally large reading area. Today the wide range of large segments having little or no image jump has reduced considerably the use of the Ultex A in the United States. Originally manufactured in plus cylinder form, it is also available in a minus cylinder design.

Note: When the term *Ultex* is used without other identification, laboratories and practitioners are referring to the Ultex A-type design.

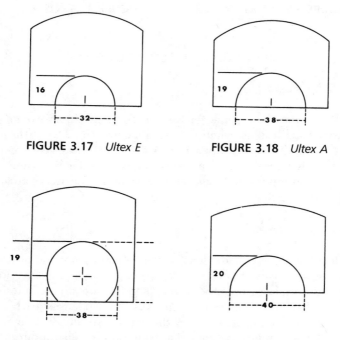

FIGURE 3.17   *Ultex E*   **FIGURE 3.18**   *Ultex A*

FIGURE 3.19   *Ultex AA*   **FIGURE 3.20**   *Ultex kingsize*

Ultex kingsize (40mm × 20mm)

The kingsize Ultex was a 40mm semicircular occupational bifocal, plus cylinder lens, manufactured in the same manner as the Ultex A and Ultex E (Figure 3.20). The factory blank results in two finished lenses, each having an optical center 20mm below the dividing line. This bifocal style is now available in a minus cylinder design but is rarely prescribed because of the large amount of image jump.

Rede-Rite (Minus Add) Bifocal (38mm × 19mm)

The Rede-Rite looks like an inverted Ultex A bifocal with the semicircular segment in the upper portion of the lens (Figure 3.21). Manufacturers identify it as a reading bifocal with a distance window. It was one of the original minus-add bifocals, but inverted segments are rarely worn today because patients prefer large-segment, occupational bifocals. The Rede-Rite may no longer be available.

High-Lite B-style (22mm Round)

This 22mm round bifocal is fashioned from one piece of high-index 1.7 glass, so the curves are flatter and the lens is considerably thinner than a comparable crown glass correction (Figure 3.22). High-Lite B-style is designed specifically as a cosmetic lens for patients needing minus 6.00D or more in the distance correction. However, because high-index is "heavy" glass and exhibits chromatic aberration, this lens is rarely prescribed.

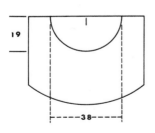
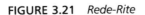
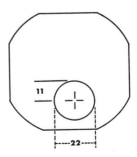

FIGURE 3.21 *Rede-Rite*   **FIGURE 3.22** *High-Lite B-style*

High-Lite A-style (38mm × 19mm)

The High-Lite A-style is an occupational, one-piece bifocal, index 1.7, designed as a cosmetically acceptable lens for high myopes (Figure 3.23). The weight of the lens, the position of the optical center, 19mm below the dividing line, and chromatic aberration severely limit its use.

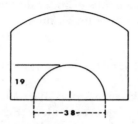

FIGURE 3.23   *High-Lite A-style*

POSITIONING THE BIFOCAL FOR CONVENTIONAL WEAR

First-time Wearer

For patients wearing bifocals for the first time, it is customary to place the segment line of straight-top and curved-top general-purpose bifocals 1mm beneath the lower lid. Most first-time wearers find this positioning satisfactory. When a patient has worn bifocals for a period of time, a slightly higher or lower position may be requested, with the segment height altered accordingly.

The round-top segment is placed a millimeter or so higher (at the lower lid) than the straight-segment designs because patients need to tilt the neck further back to utilize the maximum-width near area (through the optical center). In addition, the dividing line is not prominent and the higher positioning is not likely to be an annoyance.

PROCEDURE FOR MEASUREMENT OF BIFOCAL HEIGHT

To measure the segment top to the lower edge of the lens, the following seven steps should be performed in the order given:

1.   Place the selected frame on the patient's face.
2.   Hold the frame in the position it will occupy when the final fitting takes place.

3. With the examiner's eyes and the patient's eyes on the same level, a plastic ophthalmic ruler is placed vertically over the rims (or the lens, if it is a rimless mounting) with the zero point positioned as though it were the top of the bifocal.

4. Note the reading. If the frame shape is an aviator-type or cut off nasally, the lens must be mentally blocked into a box shape and the reading estimated to the lower lens edge (Figure 3.24).

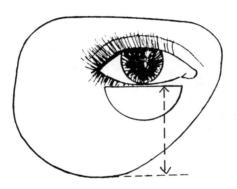

FIGURE 3.24

5. If the frame sample is the correct size and it is a wire, rimless, combination, or combination-type mounting, order the observed reading. For plastic designs add 0.5mm for light-weight and medium-weight frames, and 1mm for heavy-weight or extra-heavy-weight frames. This allows for the lens bevel that fits into the groove of the rims.

6. If the sample eyesize varies from the finished eyewear, the allowance is 1mm for each 2mm difference. For example, a 52mm eyesize frame was used to determine the bifocal height, but a 54mm eyesize is ordered. The finished lens will be 1mm wider all around, so another 1mm is added to the measurement.

7. If the patient has a hyper eye, each segment height is measured separately. Only one-half the allowance is made, however, because the difference is partially compensated for by the frame adjustment.

Example:

The right segment measures 18mm high; the left measures 20mm high. Order 18.5mm for the right lens and 19.5mm for the left. The patient with a hyper eye finds the eyewear more comfortable when angled during the final fitting in the direction of the higher eye.

There are certain conditions requiring bifocal positionings other than those described above. If the correction is used primarily for close work and is rarely worn for distance viewing, segments set 2mm or 3mm above the lower lid allow for more comfortable head/neck posture. On the other hand, patients who wear bifocals in a sunglass correction often request slightly lower segments so that the dividing line will not interfere with operating a motor vehicle.

The literature sometimes suggests that bifocals be set low when dispensed to physically challenged people, but these people should not be given bifocal lenses. Unsure of their footing when looking through plus adds, they can stumble and fall. This is a serious consideration, particularly with elderly patients who have great difficulty recovering from injuries. If in doubt, recommend two pairs: one for distance and the other for near viewing.

SEGMENT HEIGHT FOR A PREVIOUS BIFOCAL WEARER

If a patient has been wearing a bifocal correction and the case history indicates satisfaction, the new segments should occupy the same position on the face. When the patient is wearing the old glasses, note the position of the segments in relation to the lower lid. (The examiner and the patient must be on the same eye level.) With the new frame in position, place the zero point of the ruler where the top of the bifocal is desired. Proceed as previously outlined.

Note: It is critical that optically designed plastic rulers or segment measures be used. Inexpensive flexible rulers may give a false reading; metal rulers can slip and injure the patient.

Chapter 4

GLASS TRIFOCAL DESIGNS

INTRODUCTION

While bifocals fulfill a need for the presbyope by providing clear vision at distance and near, as the patient grows older the accommodative mechanism becomes less flexible. Eventually a point is reached when the bifocal segment does not provide an adequate range for both near and intermediate clear vision, a point usually noticed when the near add reaches a power of +1.75D. Clear vision at all distances can be restored by the addition of an intermediate add of less plus power than the near segment. This, then, is the advantage and the reason for the trifocal design. As the name implies, the trifocal lens has three foci: a distance correction, an intermediate power, and a near add.

Most modern trifocals are manufactured with the power of the intermediate segment 50% that of the near add. For most patients this 50% intermediate provides an excellent range of clear vision. In the few cases where this power is inadequate, the correct prescription is easily determined by a trial frame refraction. The lens can be then ordered in a design that fulfills the patient's visual requirements.

It is rarely necessary or advisable to start a beginning multifocal wearer with a trifocal correction. Bifocals are almost always adequate for first-time multifocal wearers since the add is usually relatively low in power. Furthermore, bifocals afford the patient an easier way of adjusting to the dividing line (single instead of double). In addition, optical drawbacks such as object displacement, image jump, and limitations of the near field are easier to overcome when only one segment is involved.

When the necessary add becomes +1.75D or more, it is well to consider prescribing a trifocal lens. Some patients do not require clear vision at intermediate distances and are not inconvenienced when wearing bifocals. In many cases, however, modern needs necessitate clear vision at all distances. Many patients (i.e., homemakers involved in numerous intermediate tasks such as ironing, washing, cooking, and bedmaking) are not aware of the advantages of a trifocal lens and need to have them brought to their attention. Once patients have worn trifocals they find it difficult to be satisfied with the limitations of a bifocal design.

In the fitting of trifocal lenses it is usually best to position the upper line of the intermediate segment 1mm below the pupil in normal daytime illumination (the procedure is the same as that outlined for bifocal fitting in Chapter 3, "Prescribing Modern Glass Bifocal Designs"). Most of the problems encountered in trifocal fitting stem from positioning the intermediate segment too high, resulting in a dividing line that is difficult to ignore when using the lenses for distance viewing.

To allow for an adequately sized near add, the trifocal segment for conventional wear should be at least 20mm high including the intermediate area. This height is sometimes difficult to obtain when narrow-lens/large-difference frames are prescribed. However, with the current variety of frame designs available it is always possible to find a cosmetically pleasing style into which this segment height can be fitted (occupational trifocals must be set higher than 20mm for an adequate near area).

CONSTRUCTION OF FUSED TRIFOCALS

Trifocals are manufactured in the same basic designs as bifocals. Like the bifocal, the fused form consists of a major lens blank fashioned of crown glass and segments constructed of a barium-flint combination. The countersink curve in the major blank is shaped to fit both the intermediate and near buttons. Obviously, to obtain the proper powers, the index of the near button is higher than that of the intermediate. All fused trifocals manufactured in the United States are made in minus cylinder form with the segments on the outside surface of the lens.

MATHEMATICAL COMPUTATIONS INVOLVING FUSED TRIFOCALS

For better understanding of fused bifocal designs, some of the mathematical computations involved in their manufacture were discussed in Chapter 2, "Introduction to Bifocal Lenses." Basically, the same principles are applicable to the manufacture of fused trifocal designs, the only difference being that two segment powers are involved: the intermediate add and the near add. The following additional problems relating exclusively to trifocals are given for the interested scholar (the term "Kryptok factor" remains by common usage).

PROBLEM:

A trifocal lens has a distance power of +3.00D with a near add of +3.00D and a 50% intermediate power. The index of the distance portion is 1.5; the power of the countersink curve is −4.00D; the power of the inside curve is −6.00D. Find the following:
(a) the index of the intermediate segment
(b) the index of the near segment

PROCEDURE FOR (a):

1. Determine the Kryptok factor for the intermediate.

$$K_f = \frac{F_{front} - F_{cc}}{F_{add \ (intermediate \ portion)}}$$

$$= \frac{+9.00 - (-4.00)}{+1.50}$$

$$= 8.67$$

2. Use the Kryptok factor to determine the index of the intermediate.

$$\text{Since } K_f = \frac{n_d - 1}{n_n - n_d}$$

$$n_n = \frac{(n_d - 1) + K_f n_d}{K_f}$$

$$= \frac{(1.5 - 1) + (8.67)(1.5)}{8.67}$$

$$= 1.56$$

SOLUTION TO (a):

Index of the intermediate = 1.56

PROCEDURE FOR (b):

1. Determine the Kryptok factor for the near portion.

$$K_f = \frac{F_{front} - F_{cc}}{F_{add}}$$

$$= \frac{+9.00 - (-4.00)}{+3.00}$$

$$= 4.33$$

2. Use the Kryptok factor to determine the index of the near portion.

$$n_n = \frac{(n_d - 1) + K_f n_d}{K_f}$$

$$= \frac{(1.5 - 1) + (4.33)(1.5)}{4.33}$$

$$= 1.62$$

SOLUTION TO (b):

Index of the near portion = 1.62

PROBLEM:

An ST7-25 fused trifocal with a distance prescription of $-2.00 - 0.50 \times 90$ has a near add of $+2.75D$ and a 50% intermediate. The power of the countersink curve is $-3.00D$ and of the back surface is $-8.00D$. The distance index is 1.523. Find the following:
(a) the index of the intermediate segment
(b) the index of the near segment

PROCEDURE FOR (a):

1. Determine the Kryptok factor for the intermediate.

$$K_f = \frac{F_{front} - F_{cc}}{F_{add}}$$

$$= \frac{+6.00 - (-3.00)}{+1.37}$$

$$= 6.569$$

2. Determine the index of the intermediate using the Kryptok factor.

$$n_n = \frac{(n_d - 1) + K_f n_d}{K_f}$$

$$= \frac{(1.523 - 1) + (6.569)(1.523)}{6.569}$$

$$= 1.60$$

SOLUTION TO (a):

Index of the intermediate segment $= 1.60$

PROCEDURE FOR (b):

1. Determine the Kryptok factor for the near portion.

$$K_f = \frac{F_{front} - F_{cc}}{F_{add}}$$

$$= \frac{+6.00 - (-3.00)}{+2.75}$$

$$= 3.273$$

2. Determine the index of the near portion using the Kryptok factor.

$$n_n = \frac{(n_d - 1) + K_f n_d}{K_f}$$

$$= \frac{(1.523 - 1) + (3.273)(1.523)}{3.273}$$

$$= 1.68$$

SOLUTION TO (b):

Index of the near segment $= 1.68$

FUSED TRIFOCAL DESIGNS

Straight-top Fused Trifocals.   The straight-top fused trifocal was introduced by Univis Lens Co. The design features two straight dividing lines, the upper separating the distance from the intermediate segment and the lower separating the intermediate segment from the near. The lower segment is curved in a half-round pattern. This lens is designated by two numbers, the first giving the height of the intermediate segment and the second, the maximum width of the near add.

Example:

Straight-top 7-25 (sometimes written 7/25 or 7 × 25) trifocal means the intermediate height is 7mm and the maximum width of the near segment is 25mm.

Most glass trifocals are manufactured with the intermediate segment equal to one-half the power of the near. Therefore, if the near add is +2.50D, the intermediate is +1.25D. The few designs having available varying powers will be noted when explaining the lens. The 50% intermediate is automatically supplied by the local laboratory unless otherwise specified.

Note: The straight-top designs (also called flat-top) are the most widely prescribed trifocals in the United States. Most manufacturers place the near optical center 3mm below the division separating intermediate from near.

These trifocals are distributed by major manufacturers under the following trade names:

MANUFACTURER	TRADE NAME
American Optical Corp.	Tillyer S trifocals
Shuron-Textron (formerly Shuron-Continental)	Kurova straight-top trifocals
Titmus Optical Co.	Titmus straight-top trifocals
Vision-Ease	D-style

Note: Vision-Ease took over Univis, Inc., lens operation in 1983. Univis released the lenses under the name Sentinel Trifocal Series (they had been called Nu-line, then Continuous Vision [CV] lenses).

Straight-top 6-22mm, 6-25mm, and 7-23mm

These trifocals were among the first general-purpose flat-top designs. They are rarely prescribed today because by modern standards the segment areas are limiting in size. (ST6-22 is shown in Figure 4.1.)

Straight-top 7-25

The ST7-25mm is the most widely prescribed trifocal today because its size makes it an excellent general-purpose lens (Figure 4.2). On special order, depending on the power, the intermediate segment is available with an add that is 40%, 60%, or 70% of the near, in addition to the standard 50%.

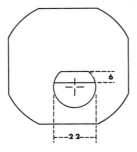

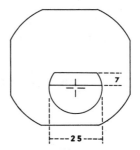

FIGURE 4.1 *Straight-top 6-22*   **FIGURE 4.2** *Straight-top 7-25*

Straight-top 7-28

Although the ST7-28 was originally designed as an occupational trifocal, its comfortable reading area has made it a lens of popular choice for the patient desiring a compromise general-purpose, large-segment multi-focal (Figure 4.3). Aside from the standard 50%, it can be specially ordered with an intermediate power that is 40%, 60%, or 70% of the near add.

Note: There is a standard D-style 6-28 available from Vision-Ease, but it is rarely prescribed.

Straight-top 7-35

The ST7-35 is a vocational "large-segment" trifocal (Figure 4.4). Because of the size of the segments, the dividing lines are relatively prominent. However, if cosmetic appearance is not a problem, this lens supplies an excellent near field for the patient who needs it. The add is also large enough to create prism at the near point by decentration. In these cases the lens is worn as a general-purpose trifocal, and, although the dividing lines are prominent, this form of correction is cosmetically supe-rior to having the prism ground into the segment. (Prism segments are available in bifocal form only. This also is a limitation.)

Straight-top 10-35

This trifocal is designed for patients needing large intermediate and near segments (Figure 4.5). It is meant as an occupational trifocal and serves best when the dividing line separating the intermediate from the distance correction is set into the pupil area. Otherwise, the patient has to maintain an uncomfortable head-back position to utilize the near segment efficiently.

Note: Vision-Ease specializes in unusual-size, custom straight-top trifo-cals. If a special combination of intermediate and near segments is desired, availability can be ascertained by querying the local laboratory.

UNUSUAL STRAIGHT-TOP DESIGNS

R-style Trifocal (6-22mm)

This trifocal features an R-style bifocal segment for the near area; the upper and lower divisions are straight lines (Figure 4.6). It is available from Vision-Ease but rarely, if ever, prescribed, since conventional gen-eral-purpose, straight-top trifocals better serve the patient's needs in design and size.

Univis Ultra CV (Glass)

This trifocal, originally manufactured by Univis, should not be confused with the plastic design having the same name and manufacturer (see Chapter 7, "Plastic Ophthalmic Lenses") but a different shape. The glass

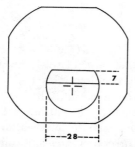

FIGURE 4.3 *Straight-top 7-28*

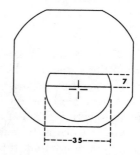

FIGURE 4.4 *Straight-top 7-35*

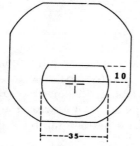

FIGURE 4.5 *Straight-top 10-35*

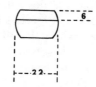

FIGURE 4.6 *R-style 6-22*

Ultra CV trifocal featured a 20mm D-shaped near add in a 30mm D-shaped intermediate area (Figure 4.7). This lens was rarely prescribed and is no longer available; patients wearing the design need to be given another trifocal style.

CURVED-TOP FUSED TRIFOCALS

Sovereign Trifocal

This design, introduced by American Optical Corp., features an intermediate segment that combines curved upper and lower borders with sharp corners. The lower segment area has the same appearance as the Sovereign bifocal. This lens incorporates a 25mm near segment with a 7mm intermediate (Figure 4.8); it is also manufactured by Vision-Ease in 7mm × 24mm. The Sovereign trifocal is a general-purpose lens that is rarely prescribed.

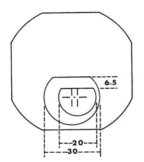

FIGURE 4.7 *Ultra CV (glass)*

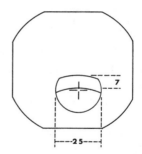

FIGURE 4.8 *Sovereign trifocal*

Panoptik Trifocal

The Panoptik trifocal, created by Bausch & Lomb, combined a 7mm intermediate segment with a 25mm near add (Figure 4.9). It featured an intermediate segment having a slightly curved top with rounded corners; the near add was D-shaped, and the two areas were separated by a straight dividing line. The lens featured a 50% intermediate when last manufactured, although in past years the intermediate power varied according to the power of the add (known as the Functional Panoptik). The lens style is no longer available.

ONE-PIECE TRIFOCALS

One-piece trifocal construction is basically similar to that of the one-piece bifocal. However, instead of two curvatures on the spherical surface of the lens, the needed power for an intermediate and near add is obtained by three changes in curvature. The "near" optical center is placed on the line dividing the intermediate from the near add.

ONE-PIECE TRIFOCAL DESIGNS

Straight-across Trifocal (Manufactured in Minus Cylinder Form)

This one-piece trifocal, distributed by American Optical Corp. under the trade name Executive trifocal, features two straight dividing lines extending across the entire lens. The intermediate area is 7mm high and has a power that is 50% of the near add (Figure 4.10). It is an excellent occupational design because the size supplies the widest segment field of any conventional trifocal. The positioning of the optical centers at the dividing lines cancels all image jump when altering fixation from one segment area to another. However, there are several disadvantages. The segments, located on the nonocular surface, have protruding shelves that tend to chip unless the patient exercises care in handling the glasses. The shelves are extremely prominent, and from a cosmetic viewpoint this trifocal is less desirable than other designs. It is best to show the patient a sample lens if appearance is a significant factor to consider. This trifocal is not desirable as a general-purpose lens. The distance area is too limiting, especially when the lens is worn while operating a motor vehicle.

Ultex T (Manufactured in Plus Cylinder Form)

The Ultex T trifocal was introduced by Continental Optical Co. The near add, 19mm round, is enclosed by a circular intermediate band 6mm to 7mm wide (Figure 4.11). Originally designed as a general-purpose trifocal, the Ultex T is rarely prescribed today. Compared to modern designs, a relatively large amount of image jump results because of the position of the optical center of the near segment (9.5mm below the lower dividing line). Furthermore, because of its small size, the near add limits the field of view. Placement of the intermediate band is such that much of its peripheral area goes unused. This kind of lens design will most likely be discontinued in the United States. It may already be no longer available.

Ultex X

This trifocal design created by Continental Optical Co. features a semi-circular near segment measuring 32mm wide on the factory blank (Figure 4.12). The 8 to 9mm intermediate circular band has an intermediate power 50% that of the near, although at one time it varied according to the add. Originally an occupational lens, it is rarely prescribed today. Considerable image jump created by the position of the near optical center (16mm below the lower dividing line) makes it undesirable in view of the superior optics of more recent trifocal designs. Although the lens was introduced in plus cylinder form, continued production of this lens will likely involve a change to a minus cylinder construction. Chances are, however, it will be discontinued in the United States.

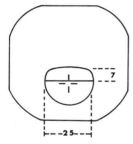

FIGURE 4.9 *Panoptik trifocal*

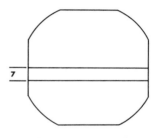

FIGURE 4.10 *Straight-across trifocal*

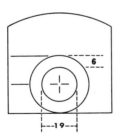

FIGURE 4.11 *Ultex T*

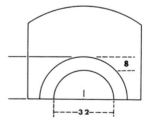

FIGURE 4.12 *Ultex X*

_____ *Chapter 5*

PRESCRIBING "INVISIBLE" MULTIFOCALS

INTRODUCTION

The association of bifocals with visual problems of middle age brought about attempts to design lenses that would be difficult to identify cosmetically as multifocals. This was inevitable. There are patients for whom the psychological, social, and occupational advantages of a youthful appearance are of prime importance.

A number of "invisible" multifocals are available; all look like single-vision lenses when the patient is viewed full face. Almost always, however, the power changes separating the near and/or intermediate areas are obvious when the head is tilted. Without exception, the major problem is the presence of unwanted cylinder, causing distorted vision when the patient looks through certain sections of the lens.

Some designs are bifocals that have an optically sound distance portion and an accurate near correction, the latter surrounded by a blur circle. Others are progressive addition-type lenses. The distance prescription is followed by power increases in a series of adds until a full near correction is reached. All such lenses have certain peripheral areas that exhibit distortion characteristics.

The earlier American-distributed variable power lens designs; the Omnifocal introduced by Univis more than three decades ago, the Progressor distributed by Titmus Optical in the late 1960s, and the Varilux 1 of the same era have been replaced by vastly improved designs. Some contemporary progressive addition lenses are detailed in this chapter.

SEAMLESS (BLENDED) BIFOCALS

Younger Seamless Bifocal

Younger Optics introduced the first seamless bifocal in 1954 and is today the world's largest manufacturer of this design (Figure 5.1). ("Seamless" is a Younger-copyrighted trade name; other manufacturers refer to the style as blended bifocals.) The dividing line that exists in other round-top bifocals is polished out, resulting in a barely perceptible blur circle. This lens, a one-piece, minus cylinder design, is available in both CR 39 plastic and glass. The glass lens, in addition to being fashioned of conventional index 1.523, can be ordered in high index, 1.7 (improving the appearance of high-power minus corrections but adding to the total weight of the eyewear).

The CR 39 plastic design is made with a 28mm-across full reading field. The width of the distorted area surrounding this field is about 3mm. The lens can be tinted any desired color.

The crown glass seamless bifocal is available with a 22mm-wide near field and a 28mm field. (The older 18mm and 20mm segment sizes have been discontinued.) The circling distorted area is about 3mm, but there are slight variations. The lower adds result in more flare-out, while the transition in the higher adds is better controlled.

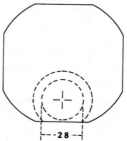

FIGURE 5.1   *Younger seamless bifocal*

In addition to a clear form, these lenses are made in Photogray Extra, pink 1 and 2, green 1, 2, and 3, and gray 3.

The High-Lite glass design, index 1.7, is made with a 22mm-wide usable near field. The surrounding blur is about 3mm wide for all prescriptions. This bifocal is available in clear and a very soft shade of pink. It is not widely prescribed because of the feeling of weight on the face and the chromatic aberration caused by the high index.

The major disadvantage of all seamless bifocals is the distortion characteristic of the blur circle. When a spherical distance correction is involved, a cylinder power is induced that is uncontrollable in both amount and axis. If the correction is a sphero-cylinder, the blur area introduces a new cylinder power at an uncontrollable axis.

Younger Optics states that the Younger Seamless bifocal is generally worn with satisfaction when it is the patient's first bifocal design. Experience has shown that the patient must also be motivated cosmetically in learning to ignore the distorted areas. The 22mm size is impractical for long periods of near work, and the addition of a separate pair of reading glasses or a ST25mm or ST28mm bifocal correction may be necessary. Whenever possible it is probably best to prescribe the 28mm size. There are patients concerned enough with cosmesis that they will wear only this kind of design for social activities.

Other Blended Bifocals

Other manufacturers distribute versions of the Younger Seamless bifocal. At present eight major manufacturers advertise usable near areas ranging from 22mm round to 28mm round. If these bifocals are desired, the local laboratory can be queried for size specifications regarding a given prescription and types of available lens materials, e.g., photochromics, high index, etc. The trade names are as follows:

MANUFACTURER	TRADE NAME
American Optical	Aolite Blended
Armorlite	Armorlite Blended
Coburn	E-Z 2 Vue
Silor	Silor Super Blend
Sola	Sola 2000
Titmus	Blenvue
Ocolite	Super Blended
Vision-Ease	Blended Segment

Fitting the Seamless (Blended) Bifocals

Unlike progressive addition lenses, blended bifocals can be fitted simply. Some manufacturers suggest measuring as though the blended lens was a round-top bifocal, usually to the top of the lower lid, and then adding 1mm (see Chapter 3, "Prescribing Modern Glass Bifocal Designs"). However, ordering the blur area to start about 3mm above the lower lid margin usually better serves the patient as it allows a more normal head/neck position for close viewing. Younger Optics even suggests the seamless be fit higher, as though it were a trifocal.

There may be a problem communicating with the local laboratory regarding segment height. The practitioner must be *specific* when ordering. If the top of the blur area is to be 1mm below the pupil margin in normal illumination (as in a trifocal), this must be stated under "special instructions." Left on their own, most technicians set the blur circle 0.5mm above and 0.5mm below the height given. For instance, the ordered height is 22mm; the blur area is 3mm wide, so 1.5mm blur is above 22mm (at 23.5mm) and 1.5mm is below. The patient, therefore, has a usable near field that is 20.5mm high.

While an accurate P.D. is important, a monocular P.D. is not necessary, making seamless bifocals the easiest "invisible" multifocals to fit. They can be more satisfactory than progressive addition lenses as the intolerant blur areas are limited in size and position, making it easier for the patient to ignore them.

CURRENT PROGRESSIVE ADDITION LENSES

Varilux (Multi-Optics)

The first progressive addition lens to have a real impact on the multifocal field was the Varilux 1. In 1951 the first steps toward developing this "invisible" multifocal featuring a gradual increase in plus add power from distance to near were begun by Société des Lundtiers of Paris, France. In 1959 marketing was started. In 1975 another version, referred to as Varilux 2, was manufactured by Essex Silor and distributed by Essilor International of France. It is currently available in the United States from Multi-Optics, a division of Essilor, and is simply called Varilux.

The Varilux 1 and Varilux feature three major optical zones. The upper portion of the lens contains the distance prescription; the intermediate zone proceeds from zero add and gradually increases in power until the near correction is reached. The remainder of the clear optical zone consists of the full near power. Vision is thus allowed to pass from distance to near in a gradual, smooth manner. Multi-Optics describes the lens as the only progressive lens having an aspheric design with the entire lower portion usable at varying distances. It has a one-piece type of construction with the changes in curvature placed on the front surface by the factory. The local laboratory grinds the finished prescription on the concave side. It can be spherical, cylindrical, prismatic, or any combination of these powers. Prism must be obtained by grinding because decentration alters the optical centers, which are factory positioned. The reading center is 13mm below and 2.5mm in from the distance optical center; the width of the progressive corridor is about 5mm.

Since the intermediate and near decentrations are predetermined, conventional multifocal segment heights are replaced by two measurements that allow the lenses to be aligned horizontally and vertically. The first of these is a monocular interpupillary distance. Accuracy is critical so a pupillometer must be used to eliminate the margin of error normally attributed to parallax. Equally as important is the distance from pupil center to the lower edge of the lens. This measurement is taken with the correct frame style and size in place while the patient fixates on a distant object and assumes natural head and eye posture. Each eye needs to be measured separately because facial asymmetry may be present. When the lens is centered according to these specifications, the progressive and full add areas will assume proper positioning when the patient converges his or her eyes.

For an adequate-size near correction the manufacturer states that the measurement from center of pupil to lower lens edge should be a minimum of 22mm. Therefore, a frame with a deep vertical shape must be selected.

The Varilux 1 exhibited an optically perfect distance portion; the distorted areas characteristic of all progressive addition lenses were concentrated in the periphery surrounding the intermediate and near corrections (Figure 5.2). The newer Varilux design spreads out the distortion, in the hope of reducing the rocking motion induced by uncontrollable cylin-

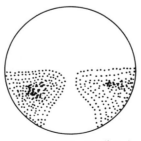

FIGURE 5.2   *Varilux 1*

drical power in amount and axis. There is some aberration in certain peripheral portions of the distance, as well as a size reduction in the optically correct near zone (Figure 5.3).

The Varilux is available in a wide range of materials. It is made in Orma CR 39 hard resin, crown glass, Photogray Extra, Photobrown Extra, a special CR 39 called UVX Light (offering complete protection against harmful ultraviolet radiations) and high-index glass for certain minus corrections.

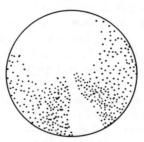

FIGURE 5.3   *Varilux*

Note: There is a Varilux Overview designed for occupational use, described in Chapter 7, "Plastic Ophthalmic Lenses."

Ultravue Progressive Power Lenses (American Optical)

The Ultravue is a CR 39 progressive addition lens manufactured by American Optical identified as a "progressive power" design. It was widely publicized to the public through full-page advertisements in prominent national magazines and on primetime television. The reference terms have become part of the terminology of progressive addition lenses. The series of add powers through which the eye travels from distance to near is called the progressive corridor. The term "optically pure" was coined to designate the areas of the lens carrying the prescribed correction, thus differentiating them from the distorted sections common to these designs.

In the Ultravue, there is a relatively wide optically pure near portion, resulting in intense peripheral distortion surrounding the add powers; this unwanted cylinder is oriented in about the 90°/180° meridians (Figure 5.4). The manufacturer feels this kind of aberration is easier to tolerate because it prevents a straight-edge object seen in the periphery from appearing curved.

The Ultravue is made only in oversize hard-resin CR 39, identified as Aolite Ultravue. This fact is advertised as a fashion advantage, enabling the lenses to be worn comfortably in larger frames. Since CR 39 lenses easily tint to any desired hue, the manufacturer promotes the availability of an infinite choice of fashion colors. The original size was an Ultravue 25 (width of near area); an Ultravue 28 design has been added.

The basic conditions necessary for a proper fit are the same as those required for aligning the Varilux: a monocular interpupillary distance and the measurement from pupil center to lower lens edge of at least 22mm. American Optical recommended the Grolman Fitting system for "absolute accuracy." This special device attaches to the front of the frame and has movable parts that center to determine the needed measurements. American Optical also made available a kit referred to as the Major Reference Point (MRP) Fitting System, advertised as a simpler means of supplying the necessary information for all progressive power lenses.

Truvision Progressive Power (American Optical)

The Truvision lens is designed by American Optical for patients needing different optical characteristics than those found in the Ultravue 25 and Ultravue 28 (Figure 5.5). There is some peripheral distortion above the 0°–180° line (similar to Varilux). The corridor is about 16mm in length and the near usable area is a circle about 20mm wide. The deeper corridor allows a more natural use of the intermediate add powers but it does mean there is more neck/head tilt to reach the widest area of the near correction.

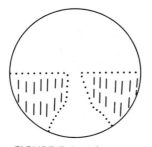
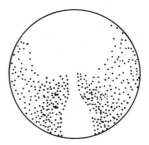

FIGURE 5.4 *Ultravue*   **FIGURE 5.5** *Truvision*

Younger 10/30™ Consecutive Power Lenses (Younger Optics)

This lens is manufactured in hard-resin CR 39 only. The first number represents the 10mm that is both the length of the consecutive transition zone and its width. The number 30 identifies the 30mm which is the effective diameter of the near area.

The Younger 10/30 is an excellent design in that the nonusable areas, present in all progressive addition lenses, are less obvious. The lateral distance area is distortion-free to the periphery; the blur zones are illustrated by the manufacturer in terms of a clock (Figure 5.6). The absence of aberration at 9 o'clock and 3 o'clock are obvious. When there is distortion in these areas, there is usually the excessive rocking motion that patients find so uncomfortable upon turning their heads.

Younger Optics reminds the practitioner that a monocular interpupillary distance is imperative and recommends that the vertical measurement be taken from the lower pupil edge to the lower lens margin (rather than from the pupil center) in order to compensate for the shorter vertical corridor.

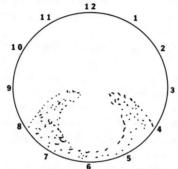

FIGURE 5.6 *Younger 10/30 consecutive lens*

Younger CPS Progressive (Younger Optics)

CPS stands for Consecutive Power Parabolic Sphere. The lens is manufactured in CR 39 plastic only and has an accurate distant prescription above the 0°–180° line. The progressive corridor is 13mm vertically. It is parabolic in nature so there is no precise horizontal width of the corridor. The size ranges from 10mm to 15mm. The distorted areas are flared compared to Younger's 10/30. The manufacturer makes this and the Younger 10/30 to meet the needs of more patients (Figure 5.7).

Unison Progressive Lenses (Vision-Ease)

Unison progressive lenses, manufactured by Vision-Ease, are reminiscent of the original Varilux 1. There is a distance portion free of astigmatism over the 0°–180° line. The advertised corridor length is 12mm, with an average 4mm width; the near area is 25mm wide (Figure 5.8). The literature emphasizes that the beginning of the progressive corridor be started at the pupil center to provide fuller distance and near areas.

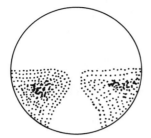
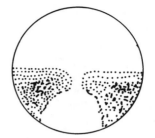

FIGURE 5.7 *Younger CPS*   **FIGURE 5.8** *Unison*

Unison is available in clear crown glass, pink, Photogray Extra, Photobrown Extra, and a CR 39 plastic having a scratch-resistant coating (SRC) on the front surface that allows for tinting any fashion color. It is also made in Lite-Gard UV, a special CR 39 lens that absorbs all harmful ultraviolet radiations below 400nm.

Continuous Vision (Vision-Ease)

The CV progressive lens is advertised as having the widest fully functional intermediate corridor of any progressive addition lens (Figure 5.9). It is 17mm in length and 11mm wide. There is an optically perfect distance area above the 0°–180° line with a near width of 20mm. The lenses are available in CR 39, clear glass, and Photogray Extra. All CR 39 CV designs are made with an "in-mold" scratch-resistant coating identified as SRC on the front surface; they can be tinted any desired color.

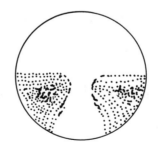

FIGURE 5.9 *CV—Continuous Vision*

Super Noline (Silor)

The Super Noline is a progressive addition lens manufactured by Silor with an accurate distant correction similar to the first Varilux. The length of the corridor is advertised at 14mm with a reading area varying from

25 to 28mm wide, depending on the lens powers (Figure 5.10). It is available in CR 39, clear glass, and some photochromic designs. There is also a special CR 39 having UVS, ultraviolet absorbing characteristics for all rays below 400nm. The scratch-resistant coated lenses are called Super Shield designs.

Note: Silor Optical is owned by Essilor, which also owns Multi-Optics, manufacturer of Varilux. The Super Noline is made to meet the needs of patients who prefer its optics to those of the Varilux.

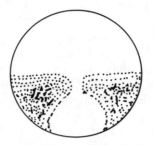

FIGURE 5.10 *Super Noline*

Natural Vue (Titmus)

This progressive lens from Titmus Optical is a relatively new design. It was first released in limited distribution during late 1984/early 1985. The Natural Vue is similar to the original Varilux 1 in that there is an accurate distance area above the 0°–180° line. The manufacturer states a relatively long, 15 to 17mm vertical corridor having a width ranging from 5 to 10mm, depending on the powers involved; the near area is 28mm wide (Figure 5.11).

The usable intermediate corridors allow a high fit capability because of the slow buildup in the progressive intermediate add powers. The suggested height from the center of the pupil to the edge of the finished lens is higher than 22mm. If the Natural Vue is fit into a frame allowing a higher measurement, the patient receives greater function when using the near correction. Natural Vue is available in CR 39 plastic (with an antiscratch coating called Cristyl Cote), clear glass, and Photogray Extra.

IMPORTANT CONSIDERATIONS REGARDING ALL PROGRESSIVE ADDITION DESIGNS

1. Extra foveal vision is disturbed by lateral aberration zones, so eye movements are restricted. There can be distur-

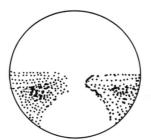

FIGURE 5.11   *Natural Vue*

bances in binocular vision. To some degree this is controlled by an accurate monocular P.D. required for all designs and by measuring vertically each eye separately from the center of the pupil or lower edge in normal illumination (see text for manufacturer's recommendation for each design) to lower lens edge. This measurement must be 22mm or higher.

Note: Each manufacturer recommends the use of a specific-design corneal reflection pupillometer. However, the basic optics are the same for all models.

2. Since the dividing lines found in conventional multifocals are absent, the lenses provide superior cosmetic benefits as well as optical advantages to the presbyope who wants clear vision in all straight-ahead positions. However, the optical distortions and reduced near field limit their use. If measurements for the progressive corridors and near areas are not given in this text, manufacturers were not specific. In all cases, manufacturers agreed there are some variations on the measurements. Clinically, it has been noted that the same design having the same prescription can have some difference in the usable-area sizes. Another problem is that all manufacturers do not use the same reference points on the lenses, so stated sizes are not as meaningful as they could be.

3. Lens measurements must be taken on the frame the patient will wear. A properly fitting bridge is critical in controlling slippage down the nose. It is best not to use frames with an obvious nasal cut (seen on most aviator designs). The best mountings for progressive addition lenses are conservative in shape, having a deep vertical dimension without being too wide horizontally.

4. A large pantoscopic angle allows the patient to "ignore" blur areas better. Lower edges of the lenses and frame should be angled close to the cheeks. A secure adjustment is very important, so straight-back temples styles should not be dispensed. Skull and comfort cable designs help hold the eyewear in place.

5. If a patient is wearing progressive addition lenses whose optics are in question, the lenses can be sent to the laboratory for identification. All manufacturers mark lenses with "signs" that can be interpreted by experts.

6. Prism cannot be obtained by decentration and must be ground into progressive addition lenses by the local laboratory.

7. While progressive addition lenses are available in a wide range of sphere, cylinder, and add corrections, there are some limits. If in doubt regarding a specific design, consult the local laboratory.

8. All manufacturers suggest an additional +0.25D add for near over that determined for a bifocal correction.

CONCLUSION

This chapter outlines the basics of the more widely used progressive addition lenses (manufacturers are promoting the term PALs), but there are over a dozen different suppliers in the United States. In 1986 "invisible" multifocals captured only about 7 to 8% of the total multifocal market. There was about an equal division between blended/seamless bifocals and PALs (statistic from the U.S. Optical Manufacturers' National Consumer Eyewear Survey).

While blended (seamless) bifocal designs appear to have found a steady market, the use of progressive addition lenses has a direct correlation between educational programs and sales figures. Seminars acquainting the eye-care professionals with advantages of specific designs are given frequently. They are a "must" if manufacturers wish the lenses to be prescribed.

For patients who will not wear multifocals "with lines," "invisible" designs are needed. While PALs are promoted for allowing clear vision at all distances, in reality, most patients seek the lenses for cosmetic reasons.

Patients requesting "invisible" multifocals are usually more satisfied when lenses are prescribed in conjunction with a utilitarian correction.

For instance, an ST28mm bifocal may be needed for an 8-hour-day job, but eyewear having more cosmetic value is preferred for after-six occasions. Others find the peripheral distortion of some progressive addition lenses unacceptable for driving a car yet welcome the lenses while shopping, since every object can be seen clearly through some portion of the lens. The gradual power change also eliminates double images that are often annoying to the conventional bifocal and trifocal wearer. When prescribing progressive addition lenses, the recommendation of a specific design depends upon professional judgment, so understanding the optics of each is imperative. The eye-care professional must be prepared to spend time teaching the patient how to use the lenses.

Note: Some manufacturers use the terms "hard structure" and "soft structure" to describe the optics of their designs. A hard-structure lens has peripheral distortion that is highly concentrated; the soft-structure design spreads out peripheral distortion, in the hope that it will be less annoying to the wearer. The illustrations used were mostly supplied by the manufacturer, but the variations due to the nature of progressive addition lenses make it impossible to always conform exactly to the accompanying text.

Chapter 6

DOUBLE-SEGMENT GLASS LENSES

INTRODUCTION

Double segment lenses are designed for presbyopic patients whose vocational and/or avocational needs involve seeing objects clearly both above eye level and at the customary reading distance. The lenses feature a lower segment having an add power almost always determined at the normal reading position and an upper segment usually focused at about arm's length. Patients most likely to benefit from double-segment lenses include eye-care professionals, pharmacists, librarians, in-store salesmen, postal clerks, and dentists. A careful case history is the best guide as to the recommendation of this lens design.

Double-segment lenses fashioned of glass (the hard-resin designs are discussed in Chapter 7, "Plastic Ophthalmic Lenses") are manufactured in both fused and one-piece construction. Almost every style has an upper add power that is a fixed percentage of the near, usually 75%. For example, if the near add is +2.50D the intermediate add is +1.87D or ¾ of the near power. The standard separation between the two segments is a fixed distance of 13 or 14mm, as determined by the manufacturer. The local laboratory can be queried for specific details.

These lenses are usually manufactured in clear and pink. The most popular, the double D-25mm, and double D-28mm, are also available in Photogray Extra, as is the Dual D-35mm design from Vision-Ease. If other intensities are needed, clear lenses can be coated with the required shade.

Since double-segment designs are relatively limited in their use, most manufacturers make available only a few styles. However Vision-Ease, the largest manufacturer of glass lenses in the United States, makes dual designs in fused segments and separations of almost any desired size. Add powers for upper and lower segments are available in most combinations. Vision-Ease stocks such a wide variety that delivery is often within the period of standard multifocals. Some specifics are mentioned here; the local laboratory can be queried for more information.

DESIGNS OF DOUBLE-SEGMENT LENSES

Straight-top Double D-25mm

This design featuring a conventional ST25mm D-style lower segment and an upper segment that is an inverted standard D-style 25mm is the most widely prescribed double-segment lens (Figure 6.1). The separation between the segments is almost always 13mm, but some manufacturers use 12mm and 14mm (check with the local laboratory for specifics). Laboratories can supply this lens in the same amount of time as any conventional multifocal with 13mm separating the two segments.

Note: Straight-top double D-22mm lenses are still available, but most manufacturers are phasing out the size.

Straight-top Double D-28mm

Two ST28mm D-style segments are placed in the same position as in the double D-25mm (Figure 6.2). The lens is for patients needing relatively

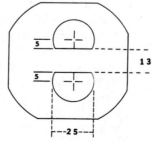

FIGURE 6.1   *Straight-top double D-25mm*

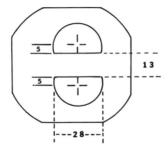

FIGURE 6.2 *Straight-top double D-28mm*

large add areas, not unusual for occupations requiring double segments. In fact, this design is rapidly approaching the popularity of the double D-25mm style. The standard separation is 13mm or 14mm, depending on the manufacturer.

DUAL D—35 SEGMENTS

This unusually wide-segment straight-top Double D design is available from Vision-Ease in crown glass and a Photogray Extra design (Figure 6.3). It is an excellent recommendation for presbyopes needing critical vision for large areas at near and overhead seeing. The standard separation between the 35mm segments is 15mm. The upper add power is not necessarily a certain percentage of the near. Specific working distances can be determined and adds ordered that fill the patient's needs. Any combination of +1.00D − +3.00D is possible. Vision-Ease makes available a pamphlet, "Ranges of Usable Clear Vision Chart For Multifocal Lenses," to aid the practitioner.

Executive Double Segment

This one-piece design introduced by American Optical Corp. features segments separated by straight lines extending from the nasal to the temporal extremities of the lens; the segments are 14mm apart (Figure 6.4). The power of the upper portion is a standard 75% of the near add. The manufacturer discourages any deviation, and it is unlikely that a double executive lens would be made with other specifications. As with all lenses of this construction, the dividing lines have a pronounced "shelf," and when high adds are involved, the outer limits tend to chip unless care is exercised in handling.

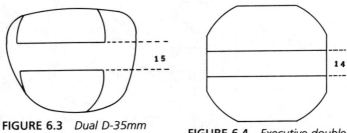

FIGURE 6.3   *Dual D-35mm*

FIGURE 6.4   *Executive double*

Double 22mm Round-top

The upper and lower segments of this fused design are 22mm round. The lower segment is conventional in appearance; the other is inverted in the upper portion of the lens (Figure 6.5). Since the widest area of each segment is 11mm from the dividing line, it is obvious a great many head/neck movements are necessary to utilize the near and intermediate areas properly. These lenses are seldom prescribed because optical performance is more advantageous in other designs.

Unusual Double-segment Designs

Lens catalogues have listed exotic double-segment lenses such as a lower Panoptik with a rounded upper segment, but they are so rare that most practitioners are familiar with them only through illustrations. At the present time, specials in glass double-segment lenses are available from Vision-Ease. The catalogue states that lenses with B- or R-style lower segments and upper segments of different D-style widths can be manufactured. Combinations with lower D-style segments and upper inverted round bifocals are custom made within a relatively short time period. However, it is almost certain that the specific needs of a patient can be satisfied with standard straight-top double-segment designs.

FITTING PROCEDURE

It is important that double-segment lenses be positioned correctly for the patient to utilize them properly. The fitting procedure outlined is offered as a guide.

1. Measure the vertical dimension of the frame selected.
2. Determine the height of the lower segment; usually the dividing line is positioned at the lower lid.

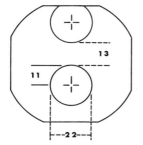

FIGURE 6.5 *Double 22mm round*

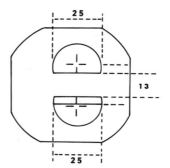

FIGURE 6.6 *Quadrifocal*

3. Add the distance separating the two segments—usually 13 or 14mm—to the height of the lower segment.

4. The remaining lens area will be the height of the upper segment. To create a comfortable, usable area of vision this measurement needs to be a minimum of 9mm. If it is not, a frame having more vertical should be dispensed. In some instances it may be feasible to position the lower segment slightly lower than usual to allow more area in the upper segment.

5. Since positioning of the two segments is critical, often minute changes in frame adjustment determine patient satisfaction. Therefore, it may be best to dispense a frame having an adjustable-pad bridge construction.

QUADRIFOCALS

It is extremely rare but possible to prescribe a lens that has an inverted bifocal segment over a trifocal design, identified as a quadrifocal (Figure 6.6). Such a lens can bring added visual efficiency to the older presbyope needing an intermediate segment as well as a bifocal for overhead seeing. Catalogues list quadrifocals available with lower segments comparable in appearance to conventional straight-top trifocals 7mm × 25mm, 7mm × 28mm, 8mm × 25mm, or 8mm × 28mm, with the upper segment an inverted straight-top D-style 25mm or 28mm bifocal. The segment separations range from 9 to 13mm. Since this is a highly sophisticated design, it is critical to query the laboratory as to availability, time, and cost factors before making a commitment to the patient. Vision-Ease is the most likely manufacturer to customize the lens to individual specifications. It is available from them in Photogray Extra for patients needing an indoor/outdoor correction.

PLASTIC
OPHTHALMIC
LENSES

INTRODUCTION

The importance of plastic lenses in a practice concerned with visual care can no longer be overlooked. Since the introduction of CR 39—the notation for hard-resin lenses—in 1947 by Armorlite, extensive research has resulted in designs often far superior to glass. About 5 years ago, polycarbonate plastic lenses further enhanced the field. Many major manufacturers in the United States are making plastic lenses and maintain consistent high quality in both prescription and plano designs.

The following discussion refers to designs that are American made/distributed because plastic lenses produced in other countries may not meet the same high standards. For instance, CR 39 lenses of a foreign design have been known to distort and yellow when placed in a hot salt pan. (Eyewear utilizing quality plastic lenses can be adjusted in the same manner as spectacles with glass lenses.) This chapter first discusses CR 39 hard-resin lenses and then compares them to polycarbonates.

ADVANTAGES OF CR 39 PLASTIC LENSES

1. **Impact resistant.** Plastic lenses offer more ocular protection than those of a glass design. While chemically tempered lenses may have the same impact-resistant quality as glass (see Chapter 10, "Impact-Resistant [Safety] Lenses"), if a glass lens breaks, there is a possibility of splinters "kicking back" and imbedding into the eye and adnexa. It is extremely rare for a CR 39 lens to shatter, and when it does, the breakage almost always consists of large fragments unlikely to inflict serious injury.

2. **Light weight.** Hard-resin CR 39 lenses are approximately 50% lighter than those constructed of glass, assuming the same eye size and prescription. This characteristic is particularly important when large frames are dispensed. It is difficult for patients to be comfortable wearing glass lenses measuring greater than 52mm horizontal box diameter. Patients who have recently undergone rhinoplasty (nose surgery) should be prescribed plastic lenses. The bridge usually swells under the slightest pressure; this condition often lasts for about a year. If the nasal bones were broken or extensive surgery was involved, sensitivity may last a lifetime. Elderly patients whose epithelial tissue has lost its elasticity are acutely aware of pressure and are more comfortable wearing plastic lenses.

3. **Less tendency to fog.** When a patient goes from a cold to warm environment, CR 39 plastic lenses are less likely to fog than are those made of glass. This is advantageous for patients engaged in occupations where a change in temperature occurs with frequency (e.g., a butcher), although patients should be told that fogging is reduced and not eliminated. If fogging continues to be a problem, contact lenses are often the ideal solution.

4. **Can be tinted any color to give any effect.** While practitioners may prefer uniform tinting on a CR 39 lens, coloring can be easily varied if desired. Gradient shading, with the upper portion of the lens having a darker color fading into a softer hue, and the use of two soft colors in juxtaposition are extremely popular fashion looks. If a minus correction is tinted the intensity of a suntone, the characteristic myopic rings disappear. While the lighter shades are not quite as effective in reducing internal reflections, they

vastly improve the cosmetic value of a lens compared to its clear form.

5. **Absorb ultraviolet radiation.** Overexposure to intense ultraviolet radiation can lead to pathological involvements of the eye and its adnexa. Some patients are photophobic under fluorescent lighting. Quality-plastic CR 39 lenses absorb all ultraviolet (UV) to 350nm. There are also available lenses with UV-absorption capabilities to 400nm. These are especially recommended for aphakes who have had conventional surgery as the retina is exposed to an abnormal amount of radiation when the ocular crystalline lens is removed. While the newer procedure involves an implant lens (patients are called pseudophakes) having UV absorbers, most practitioners provide a UV-absorbing spectacle lens for added protection. (The older implant procedure did not use a UV-absorbing lens.)

Note: A lens called Full Spectrum, which does not absorb UV rays, is available from Armorlite. However, it is not used to fill a prescription unless specifically requested.

POSSIBLE DISADVANTAGES OF CR 39 PLASTIC LENSES

The advantages of these lenses far outweigh the disadvantages but there are a few considerations requiring patient counseling. Most problems can be eliminated by the simple precautions explained here.

1. **Less scratch-resistant than glass.** For years the relative softness of the lens' surfaces made some practitioners hesitant in recommending CR 39 hard-resin. Modern advances in technology have resulted in lenses that stay scratch-free with very little care. They should be cleaned by holding under running water, preferably warm, to wash away dust that may act as an abrasive and then dried with a soft tissue or cloth. For emergency use, plastic lens cleaners are available, but they may leave an annoying film. Patients need to be cautioned against laying the eyewear down with the lenses touching a hard or rough surface. Because of the popularity of hard-resin CR 39, cases that completely envelop the eyewear with a soft, silky lining or a velvety-textured fabric are easily available. Note: Within recent years, it has been possible to order

special coatings that make CR 39 lenses highly scratch resistant. Their practical use is discussed in Chapter 8, "Ophthalmic Lens Coatings."

2. **Lack of an absorber for infrared radiations.** When absorbers for infrared (IR) are used in the manufacturing procedure, they give prescription plastic lenses a milky look. Research to develop a clear absorber is a major goal of ophthalmic scientists. If a patient is exposed consistently to bright or reflected sunlight or works around molten glass/metal, tinted-glass designs having clearly designated absorption curves should be recommended.

Note: Plano CR 39 lenses in suntints that absorb UV and IF are available. They are discussed in Chapter 9, "Prescribing Absorptive Lenses."

3. **Transmission curves for tints are rarely released.** Plastic lenses are tinted by dipping into color solutions, the formulas for which depend on the dye used by the local laboratory. As a result, rarely if ever does an optical company make available charts showing transmission and absorptive properties of the visible spectrum for the various hues of CR 39.

Note: UV/IF absorption/transmission is determined by absorbers used in the manufacturing process. Curves for these potentially harmful radiations can be obtained by querying specific manufacturers.

4. **Cosmetic appearance of clear minus and prism lenses.** Since the index of CR 39 lenses is 1.49 as compared to 1.523, the standard for crown ophthalmic glass, they are thicker for any given prescription. While this is rarely a problem when plus lenses are involved, the edges of high minus and prism lenses can be relatively pronounced. Because plastic does not have the transparency of glass, the opaque look of the bevel further emphasizes the problem. The hide-a-bevel method of edging lenses is an excellent aid, and advances in optical equipment make it possible to use this procedure on CR 39 regardless of size or prescription. Tinting the lenses is a cosmetic plus because any hue, even the palest tone, helps cover the "whitish" edges.

Note: Sometimes a color edge coating that blends with the frame improves cosmesis. Edge coatings are discussed in Chapter 8, "Ophthalmic Lens Coatings."

5. **Bitoric effect in rimmed frames.** Pressure of the mounting against CR 39 lenses causes a change in their form resulting in a bitoric effect (cylinder on both surfaces). This problem cannot be eliminated with rimmed mountings because a lens mounted loosely will fall out of the frame. However, the bitoric effect can be limited to 1.00D, which conforms to the optical standards set by the American National Standards Institute (ANSI). The toricity should be checked by clocking both surfaces with a lens gauge upon receiving the eyewear from the laboratory. It is interesting to note that limited bitoric effect in compliance with ANSI is always the case when hard-resin CR 39 lenses are mounted in optyl frames. The problems that arise tend to involve only metal and nylon mountings.

SPECIAL NOTES CONCERNING CR 39 LENSES

Not all laboratory procedures applicable to glass lenses are suitable for hard-resin CR 39.

1. Since plastic tints are not standardized, if a single tinted lens is ordered, the other must be sent to the laboratory for a color match.

2. Resurfacing a plastic lens to remove scratches or to make changes in the power is impractical. Most laboratories will not alter CR 39, cataract lenses being the exception because of high replacement cost.

3. Before attempting to adjust eyewear utilizing hard-resin lenses, the lens origin should be ascertained. Those of foreign manufacture may discolor or become distorted when subjected to a frame-heating device.

4. At one time deeply tinted plastic lenses were not as attractive as their glass counterparts. The brown tones tended to have a reddish cast; the gray tints could appear purplish. These problems no longer exist when skilled technicians use the vastly improved lens dyes.

5. Provided the surfaces are scratch free, quality CR 39 can be bleached and retinted satisfactorily if the color fades or another shade is desired. Drastic color changes/effects are possible.

AVAILABILITY OF HARD-RESIN CR 39 DESIGNS

The range of CR 39 designs is almost comparable to that of glass lenses. Certainly, every conventional multifocal as well as single-vision designs are now available in both CR 39 and glass. In addition, there are some special designs, particularly cataract lenses (see Chapter 11, "Lenses for Special Uses"), fashioned exclusively of hard-resin CR 39. Major manufacturers use the following trade names when distributing hard-resin CR 39 plastic lenses:

MANUFACTURER	TRADE NAME
American Optical Corp.	Aolite
Signet Armorlite	Armorlites
Silor	Orma
Optical Radiation	Orcolite
Titmus Optical Co.	Cristyl
Vision-Ease	Unilite
Shuron-Textron	Kurovalite
Bausch & Lomb, Inc.	formerly Ortholite (B&L has ceased production of prescription plastic lenses.)

Most local laboratories stock single-vision spherical corrections ranging in power from plano through +20.00D, and from −0.25D to −25.00D in 0.25D steps. Plano-cylinder and sphero-cylinder lenses are stocked in minus cylinder form with the former usually ranging in power from 0.25 D to 6.00D. Stocked sphero-cylinder lenses depend upon the combination of powers. Any single-vision prescription available in glass can be ground in CR 39 by the local laboratory.

BIFOCAL DESIGNS

Plastic multifocals are one-piece lenses ground in minus cylinder form. All popular bifocal styles available in glass have an optical counterpart in hard-resin CR 39.

One of the most welcomed developments in the hard-resin field is the availability of oversize blanks in a wide range of bifocal and trifocal designs. Many presbyopes are older patients who cannot tolerate the heaviness of glass. Fashion hues, another important part of contemporary eyewear styling, are easily applied to bifocal plastic lenses. When a gradient tint has the color change at the dividing line, the effect is often that of fashion eyewear without any loss of cosmetic value.

Straight-top (Flat-top) 22mm Bifocal

The basic concept of a segment having a straight division with a rounded lower area and a segment optical center 5mm below the dividing line has been the most popular in the United States (Figure 7.1). The ST22mm bifocal, one of the original sizes, has outlived its usefulness and been replaced by the ST25mm and the ST28mm, which provide a wider reading area while retaining the same optical principles. Most manufacturers have discontinued the size but it is available from Vision-Ease.

Note: The ST23mm CR 39 bifocal available some years back is no longer manufactured.

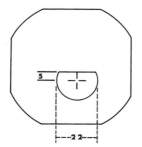   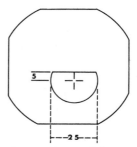

FIGURE 7.1 *Straight-top 22*   **FIGURE 7.2** *Straight-top 25*

Straight-top 25mm Bifocal

The flat-top 25mm design is the most popular bifocal style in the United States (Figure 7.2). The near area is large enough to read open pages of a book at a glance, while the distance prescription surrounding the segment provides adequate space for far viewing (e.g., driving a car). Oversize CR 39, ST25mm lenses are available for most prescriptions, so the practitioner can dispense frames having an eyesize of up to 56 or 58mm.

Straight-top 28mm Bifocal

Although the ST28mm segment was originally designed as an occupational bifocal for patients needing a relatively large near area, its popularity makes this an excellent general-purpose lens (Figure 7.3). The segment is very compatible to the appearance of large frames. Patients who do a great deal of close viewing yet do not wish to invest in separate eyewear for occupational use, particularly enjoy flat-top 28mm segments.

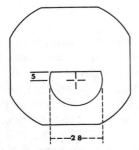
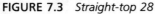
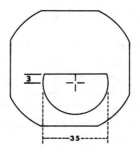

FIGURE 7.3 *Straight-top 28*   **FIGURE 7.4** *Straight-top 35*

Straight-top 35mm Bifocal

Answering the need for an occupational bifocal that has more cosmetic value than the straight-across segment, a number of manufacturers have made the flat-top 35mm available in CR 39 blanks (Figure 7.4). The finished lens should easily cut to a 56mm horizontal box measurement in most prescriptions if desired. The optical center of the near segment is 3mm below the dividing line.

Straight-top 40mm Bifocal

This occupational lens, developed by Armorlite, is available only in a plastic design. The ST40mm was introduced for the patient desiring an exceptionally large near field yet objecting to the appearance of the "shelves" conspicuous in the Executive-style bifocal (Figure 7.5). Patients accustomed to the full near field of a straight-across segment find it fills their needs while improving cosmetic value. One of the reasons is the similarity in optics. The optical center of both designs is at the line separating the distance from the near areas.

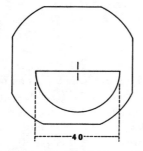
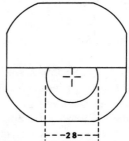

FIGURE 7.5 *Straight-top 40*   **FIGURE 7.6** *Slab-off straight-top 28*

Slab-off Straight-top Bifocal

Slab-off (bicentric) grinding is the best method of correcting for vertical imbalance at near. At one time patients needing such a correction could have it only in glass. Today expert optical technicians can incorporate most bicentric corrections in hard-resin straight-top bifocals. Practitioners often recommend the ST25mm, although the slab-off line is less obvious when it coincides with the dividing line of the flat-top 28mm (Figure 7.6).

Note: Younger Optics has introduced a reverse slab-off in CR 39. It is discussed in Chapter 13, "Vertical Imbalance at the Reading Level."

Executive-type Bifocal

This lens with the segment area extending from the temporal to the nasal-edge extremities offers the widest reading area possible in a bifocal design (Figure 7.7). At one time it was often impossible to prescribe oversize CR 39 Executive bifocals because of the manufacturer's limitations. Although this condition has been rectified, it must be kept in mind that the larger the lens and/or the higher the add power, the more obvious the outer extremities of the segment. Because of the cosmetic disadvantages, intensified by the thickness problem, the patient should see a sample before ordering.

Round-top 22mm Bifocal

The round-top 22mm segment has enjoyed popularity for many years as the least visible of the optically sound bifocal designs (Figure 7.8). While the position of the optical center at 11mm below the top of the dividing line necessitates unnatural tilting back of the head to reach the widest area, patients motivated by cosmesis learn to live with the limitations. Times have changed and mature women working outside the home often find themselves in jobs requiring maximum visual effi-

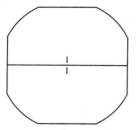

FIGURE 7.7 *Straight-across bifocal*

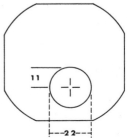

FIGURE 7.8 *Round-top*

ciency. They tend to seek cosmetic value from the styling of the frame and fashion tinting of the lenses rather than segment style. For the patient still wanting this inconspicuous bifocal, a fashion hue on the entire lens results in a barely visible segment, particularly in the lower add powers.

Ultex-style Bifocal

While the Ultex A, half-moon bifocal (38mm across at the lowest area of the segment) has a segment optical center 19mm below the dividing line, which causes considerable image jump, some older patients who have worn the lens for decades still request it (Figure 7.9). As a result the design is made in plastic minus cylinder form. Since the original glass Ultex A was in a plus cylinder form, the patient may experience a few problems due to base-curve changes. However, the reduction of meridional astigmatism in minus cylinder lenses makes them more desirable, and they should prove satisfactory after a short adjustment period. Prescription and blank-size availability need to be checked with the local laboratory because there is relatively little demand for A-style segments.

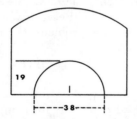 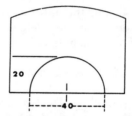

FIGURE 7.9   *Ultex A-style*   **FIGURE 7.10**   *Wide seg-40*

Wide Seg-40 Round (40mm × 20mm)

The positioning of the optical center of this segment, 20mm below the dividing line, is comparable to that of the glass King-Size Ultex (Figure 7.10). The high amount of image jump limits its use; large straight-top segments that have optical centers close to or at the dividing line are preferable occupational bifocals.

Curved-top with Sharp Corners

The glass counterpart is the Tillyer Sovereign, and although several plastic bifocals similar in appearance have been distributed in the United States, they are rarely seen. The Orma-Arc by Silor (France), having a 26mm width, was the most popular, but it is no longer available here

(Figure 7.11). American Optical's Aolite C-25 Sovereign had very limited distribution.

TRIFOCAL DESIGNS.

There are now available CR 39 trifocal designs that meet the needs of presbyopes requiring specific-size intermediate segments. Like bifocals, they are manufactured in one-piece minus cylinder form. The standard near adds range in power from +1.50D to +3.00D, depending on the design (the local laboratory can be queried for specifics), with a standard intermediate power that is 50% of the near addition. Vision-Ease also makes several designs with intermediate segment powers 40%, 60%, and 70% of the near add. They are discussed in this chapter.

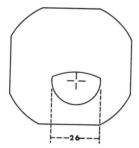

FIGURE 7.11   *Orma-Arc*

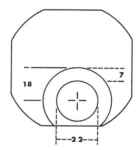

FIGURE 7.12   *Round-top trifocal*

Round-top Trifocal

The round-top trifocal features a 22mm round near segment surrounded by an intermediate circular band of 7mm (Figure 7.12). It was the first trifocal made in CR 39. Since the straight-top designs offer more efficiency and optical value, this lens is rarely seen today.

Straight-top (Flat-top) 7mm × 25mm Trifocal

This is the most widely prescribed trifocal in both glass and plastic. Straight dividing lines separate the intermediate segment from the distance area and the intermediate from the near. The intermediate is a band 7mm high; the near segment is a straight-top D-style bifocal (rounded lower extremities). Adequate viewing areas are provided for most patients, and a relatively pleasing cosmetic appearance is maintained (Figure 7.13).

Until recently, this CR 39 design was made only with the standard 50% intermediate segment power. Now, as in the case of the glass counterpart, Vision-Ease makes available the ST7-25 with an intermediate power that can be ordered 40%, 60%, or 70% of the near add.

Note: The original ST6-22 CR 39 trifocal has been phased out because of the limited size segment areas.

Straight-top 7mm × 28mm

Comparable in appearance to the ST7-25 trifocal, the use of this lens is increasing (Figure 7.14). Many patients enjoy the near area; 28mm allows for an exceptionally wide, comfortable field.

In addition to the standard 50% intermediate power, Vision-Ease supplies the design with an intermediate power that is 40%, 60%, or 70% of the near add.

Note: The ST7-25 and ST7-28 plastic trifocals are appropriate designs when a bicentric correction is indicated. The slab-off line is customarily placed to coincide with the division between the intermediate and near segments (Figure 7.15).

Straight-top 7mm × 35mm

Designed for the patient needing an exceptionally wide near area, the 35mm near segment is a popular occupational trifocal (Figure 7.16).

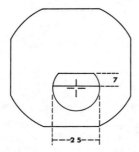

FIGURE 7.13   *Straight-top 7-25*

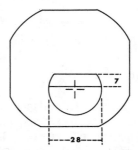

FIGURE 7.14   *Straight-top 7-28*

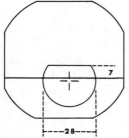

FIGURE 7.15   *Slab-off straight-top 7-28*

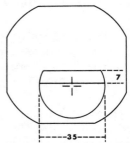

FIGURE 7.16   *Straight-top 7–35*

As with all large-segment lenses, the dividing lines are relatively pronounced but not as obvious as those in the straight-across trifocal design. The lens can also be used for slab-off corrections.

DATALITE TRIFOCAL FOR VDT USERS

In 1986 Vision-Ease released the Dataline trifocal for wear at video display terminals (VDTs). The lens is available in hard-resin CR 39 only. The near add is a ST35mm segment; the intermediate segment measures 14mm high, giving an excellent vision area at the distance most VDTs are placed (Figure 7.17). The power, 66% of the lower add, was determined by research to give the best intermediate acuity. The lens exhibits UV-absorbing characteristics. Color compatible to the in-mold scratch-resistant coating applied at the factory level can be ordered if the patient needs additional protection from glare.

Straight-across (Full-segment) Trifocals

This lens looks like an Executive glass trifocal. Both the near and intermediate segments extend to the extremities of the lens blank with the intermediate band measuring 7mm high (Figure 7.18). The distance correction thus is limited to the upper portion of the lens. It is strictly a vocational design for patients needing unusually large and/or wide intermediate and near segments. Cosmesis is poor because of the obvious "shelves" of the dividing lines.

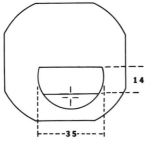

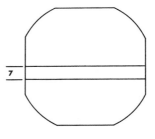

FIGURE 7.17   *Datalite trifocal—VDT*   **FIGURE 7.18**   *Straight-across trifocal*

Sola E/D Trifocal (Sola Worldwide)

As the initials *E/D* imply, the Sola E/D trifocal features an Executive-style intermediate segment that extends from the temporal to the nasal extremities of the lens and surrounds a 25mm straight-top D-style reading segment (Figure 7.19). It is made in plastic only. Manufactured in Europe, it has become increasingly difficult to obtain in the United States.

Univis Ultra CV (Continuous Vision)

This Ultra CV trifocal had a distinctive design best visualized by looking at Figure 7.20. The near segment is a 24mm D-style positioned inside an intermediate area measuring 28mm at the widest point.

Univis has discontinued all lens production, and no other manufacturer makes the design. Patients wearing this lens need to be changed to another general-purpose trifocal. The ST7-25mm or ST7-28mm should prove satisfactory.

Note: A glass trifocal having the same name, Ultra CV, but a slightly different shape was also manufactured by Univis. It, too, is no longer available.

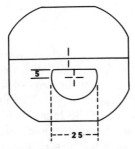

FIGURE 7.19   Sola E/D (Executive/D-style segments)

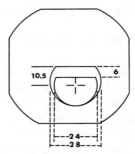

FIGURE 7.20   Univis Ultra CV— CR 39

DOUBLE-SEGMENT OCCUPATIONAL LENSES

Double-segment lenses, characterized by upper and lower adds separated by the distance prescription, are designed to give the patient an add power for overhead seeing. People whose occupations require this kind of clarity include pharmacists, dentists, and showroom salespeople. The distance area is limited to the separation between the two segments (the standard is 13mm or 14mm, depending on the design), so these lenses are prescribed in addition to conventional eyewear. The procedure for positioning double segments is explained in Chapter 6, "Double-Segment Glass Lenses."

Double D (ST25mm Segments)

The double D-25mm lens is the choice of many practitioners for the patient requiring this type of design; the segment areas for both overhead and near viewing are ST25mm D-style bifocals (Figure 7.21). The usual separation between the two is a standard 13mm, with the upper segment power 75% of the near add. However, Vision-Ease makes a wide range in combinations of addition powers and separations in the Dual D-25mm design. The local laboratory should be queried for details if the patient history indicates a special need.

Double D (ST28mm Segments)

This double D-28mm lens is increasingly the choice for occupational use (Figure 7.22). The segment areas for both overhead and near viewing are ST28mm D-style bifocals. The usual separation between the two is a standard 13mm with the upper segment power 75% of the near add. However, a trade-named "DD-Double Seg Occupational" by Younger Optics was recently introduced in an exclusive-type flat-top 28mm CR 39. It has a standard 14mm separation between the two 28mm segments and is available with two possible combination add powers. One features the same add for the upper and lower segments (e.g., bottom add, +2.00D; upper segment add, +2.00D). The other possibility is a top segment power approximately 62% of the power of the bottom segment (e.g., near add, +2.00D; upper segment, +1.25D).

Executive-style Double Full Segment

This Executive-style lens has the upper and lower segments extending from the temporal to the nasal extremities of the lens blank with the distance power a vertical band 14mm high (Figure 7.23). The upper

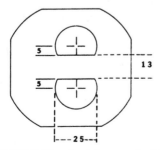

FIGURE 7.21 *Straight-top double D-25mm*

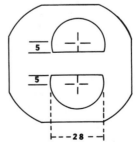

FIGURE 7.22 *Straight-top double D-28mm*

segment has an intermediate power 75% of the near. The lens gives the widest field possible for intermediate and near viewing, but a cosmetic problem lies in the prominence of the dividing lines.

Double Round (25mm Segments)

These designs are listed in current lens catalogues as available with segment separation of 14mm. However, the patient needs to hold the head and neck awkwardly to reach the widest area of the segments (through the optical centers). The positioning of the optical centers, 12.5mm from the dividing line, also introduces considerable image jump (Figure 7.24). Almost always, the patient is better served with a Double D-25mm lens.

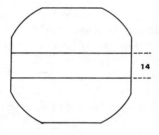

FIGURE 7.23   *Executive double*

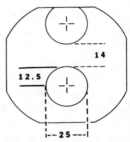

FIGURE 7.24   *Double 22mm round*

"INVISIBLE" MULTIFOCALS

There are available many "invisible" multifocals with an absence of dividing lines between the various power changes in CR 39 lenses. This is true for both seamless/blended and progressive addition lenses. They are discussed in Chapter 5, "Prescribing 'Invisible' Multifocals." However, a special design released in 1986 by Multi-Optics called Varilux Overview is discussed here because its use is the same as a double-segment lens.

Varilux Overview

The lower part of the lens is a normal Varilux progressive addition. The upper area carries a 41mm bifocal shaped like a half-moon. The distance between the central fitting cross and the segment edge is 9mm. The upper add power is always 0.50D less than the full add (e.g., for a +2.00D maximum near, the add at the top is +1.50D) (Figure 7.25). The manufacturer recommends the Varilux Overview for technicians, mechanics, painters, and librarians, but while the upper usable segment is excellent, there is peripheral distortion in other parts of the lens. Professional judgment and a careful case history is important before prescribing. To give an adequate upper area, a deep frame pattern that allows 10mm to 12mm segment height is necessary. Probably the upper segment division is best placed at the upper edge of the pupil in normal illumination.

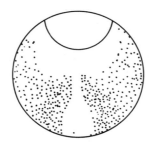

FIGURE 7.25 *Varilux Overview*

POLYCARBONATE PLASTIC LENSES

These relatively new plastic lenses have a high index of 1.586, making them more attractive than hard-resin CR 39 (index 1.49). They are the safest/strongest lenses available and also the lightest in weight. They filter all harmful UV radiations.

Within the past few years, polycarbonate plastic lenses have made a great impact on the eyewear field. Many manufacturers make the lens available, and while some claims differ, these are the basic advantages:

1. They are thinner than CR 39, with an advertised range of 15% to 20%. This is especially noted in the reduction of thick-edged high minus lenses.

2. They are lighter than glass by 55% to 60% and lighter than CR 39 by about 10%.

3. They are the safest lenses available: 25 times more impact resistant than hard-resin CR 39.

4. They block 99% to 99.9% of harmful UV radiations.

5. They are highly scratch and abrasion resistant because of coatings applied on both surfaces (this must be done by a high quality manufacturer).

There are disadvantages. While all polycarbonates are made of the same material, there is a difference in quality because of the methods of manufacturing and processing procedures. Some offer much better abrasion resistance than others. All high-index lenses exhibit chromatic aberration, particularly noticed in the periphery (dispensing the smaller frames currently in style helps this problem). Laboratories may have difficulty producing attractive suntints.

Although the available prescription range is expanding, there are serious limitations compared to CR 39. Spherical corrections include ±10.00D with a considerable smaller range in sphero-cylinder combinations. Cylindrical powers are limited. ST25mm and ST28mm bifocals are available in a smaller range of powers; so is a ST7-25mm trifocal. Many more lens designs are planned for release in the near future, so local laboratories should be contacted frequently for updated information.

As the coating systems improve and the prescription range expands, these lenses will capture a high percentage of the ophthalmic market. While all local laboratories do not have the equipment to fabricate these lenses, more are offering this service.

Gentex Corporation is the market leader. Included among other manufacturers who supply polycarbonate lenses are Vision-Ease (trade name Herculens), Omega Group (Lite Style), Eye-Kraft Optical, Inc. (Eyelite XT 30), and Associated Optical (Maxilite).

YOUNGERLITE HIGH-INDEX PLASTIC LENSES

Younger Optics has recently released high-index plastic lenses advertised as combining most of the advantages of polycarbonates with the workability of CR 39. Called Youngerlite, its 1.56 index makes for very attractive minus lenses. Its main advantage over polycarbonate lenses lies in the fact that the local laboratory can use standard hard-resin equipment and methods to fabricate the prescriptions (polycarbonates need special equipment for processing). There is less chromatic aberration because of the lower index. Youngerlite absorbs to 380nm UV radiations, which is adequate protection against these harmful rays.

There can be a problem in obtaining a tinted Youngerlite lens. The front surface has a hard, nontintable coating, so coloring must take place on the back surface. The lenses sometimes come out with a slight variation in shading regardless of the appropriate dye bath and care of the optical technician.

PRESCRIBING CR 39 LENSES VS POLYCARBONATES

Undoubtedly, polycarbonate lenses will be used in the future for all safety eyewear. They offer the best protection for children needing a correction most or all waking hours. High myopes appear exceptionally pleased with the appearance of their eyewear when polycarbonate lenses are prescribed.

At present, hard-resin CR 39 lenses offer a wider prescription range. Any desired multifocal style is available in CR 39, whereas the polycarbonate designs are extremely limited. In addition, CR 39 lenses can be ordered with UV-absorption capabilities to 400nm (comparable to polycarbonates). It will be a while before polycarbonate lenses are recommended as often as CR 39, but high-index material appears to be the future of lens designs.

Chapter 8

OPHTHALMIC LENS COATINGS

INTRODUCTION

Perhaps the most remarkable addition to the lens design field during the past few years is the development and increased use of coatings applied to surfaces of glass and plastic lenses. They can enhance fashion tinting, are available in colors that absorb radiations harmful to the eye, and are applied in antireflection form so that direct and reflected light is less bothersome to the wearer of glasses. This chapter discusses currently used coatings for glass and plastic lenses.

COATINGS FOR GLASS LENSES

There are available several types of coatings that offer specific advantages to the patient when applied to glass lenses. These coatings are not to be confused with the coatings for hard-resin CR 39 and polycarbonate lenses that result in a hard, abrasion-resistant surface (discussed later).

The glass coating most commonly prescribed is an antireflection layer applied to both surfaces of the lens. The process makes it possible to eliminate approximately two-thirds of the reflections normally noted on crown lenses and about three-fourths of that ordinarily seen on high-index glass.

Since a lens is visible because of reflected light from its surfaces, an antireflection coating offers several cosmetic advantages. Coated lenses are so clear that they often appear almost invisible. The eye area is seen in better perspective, thus allowing for more expressive interest in the face.

Lens coatings for glass are also available in a wide variety of colors. These tints are applied either to the front or the back surface of the lens or to both surfaces, depending on the professional judgment of the manufacturer. To reduce reflections, an antireflection coating is usually applied over the color coating.

A coating of a protective nature, sometimes referred to as a permanent layer, is also available. It is placed over color and antireflection coatings to help keep them intact.

ANTIREFLECTION COATINGS

When a beam of light strikes a clear ophthalmic glass lens, light transmission is about 92%. The remaining 8% is lost through reflections from the front and back surfaces of the lens. Although this loss of light can result in a slight decrease in visual acuity, the problem usually encountered by the patient is awareness of annoying reflections.

An antireflection coating is composed of ¼ of a wavelength of magnesium fluoride. While it is a physical impossibility to coat a lens to be completely free of a tinge of color, the index of magnesium fluoride (about 1.36) allows a crown lens to appear almost colorless when applied by a skilled technician. However, the index is a little too high for best results when high-index lenses are involved, and the lenses may have a slight purplish hue. To counteract this effect, most laboratories apply a thin "straw" film achieved by stopping just short of the application of ¼ of a wavelength. This slightly golden cast is almost always preferable to the purplish look.

Some practitioners recommend an antireflection coating on all glass lenses. However, the following patients may benefit more than others when this coating is used:

1.   Patients concerned about the annoyance of reflected light when driving at night. In dim illumination, reflections of bright objects such as oncoming headlights are often manifested as double images. In many cases, the driver's judgment as to distance and other vision-related factors is adversely affected. An antireflection coating provides

a more comfortable environment, thereby making night driving safer.

2. Patients wearing a correction of minus 2.00D and greater. The presence of myopic rings is a major cosmetic disadvantage with minus lenses. These internal reflections are considerably reduced with the use of an antireflection coating.

3. Patients wearing high-power plus lenses. When plus lenses are worn, the ghost images reflected from the lens surfaces, although rather vague, are relatively large and can be very annoying. An antireflection coating reduces this source of irritation, as well as improving the appearance of the eyewear.

4. Patients wearing high-power prism lenses. If the prism power is high enough for a noticeable difference in edge thickness to be present, the lenses are a cosmetic problem. Since reflections from the surfaces of a prism are also pronounced, coating the lenses helps their appearance.

5. Any patient wearing glasses who is concerned about ghost images and/or light reflections. There are sensitive patients who are bothered by lens reflections even when the correction is low in power. Often they are wearers of multifocals, particularly concerned about reflections at the segment dividing lines. While some manufacturers attempt to solve the problem by coating the dividing lines of fused segments, the best results are achieved when the entire lens is treated with an antireflection coating.

Note: Antireflection coatings are sometimes confused with pink tints. Somehow, there is a mistaken conception that they solve the same problem, probably because both are recommended for reduction of glare. An antireflection coating allows more light to enter the eye; a tinted lens reduces light transmission. If there is a desire to reduce both lens reflections and light transmission, a pink no. 2 tint with an antireflection coating can be recommended. Light transmission through such a lens is approximately 88%.

While antireflection coatings are available from hundreds of optical suppliers, it is the Hoya Lens manufacturer who has concentrated on the promotion of these coatings. While many companies use ordinary single-layer or two-layer coatings, Hoya developed a unique multi-layered coating that allows over 99% of light to go through a clear lens (compared to about 96% with two-layer coatings and 92% with noncoated clear glass lenses). Called Hoya 99 Multicoated Lens, it eliminates the "glassiness" of a clear lens, making it almost invisible. Thus, the eye area is seen more naturally. Interestingly, although the difference in percentage of light transmission seems slight, in actual use patients report improved vision and lowered eye fatigue. Other multilayered antireflection coatings are currently available and the local laboratory can be queried for details.

Some manufacturers may use from three to nine layers, but efficiency is related not to the number of layers but to the selection of materials for refractive index, the thickness with which the layers are applied, and adherence capability to the previous layer.

COLOR COATINGS

Metal oxide coatings in almost any desired color can be applied to glass lenses. There are several advantages to ordering lenses tinted by this method. When a suntint prescription other than plano is involved, glass lenses manifest a color difference from center to edge. This difference is barely perceptible in prescriptions under ±2.00D. When the prescription is over ±4.00D, the difference is almost always obvious enough that a method of color control is necessary (see Chapter 9, "Prescribing Absorptive Lenses"). One of these methods involves coating the lenses the desired shade. Since the color is applied evenly over the lens surface (unless otherwise ordered), it is always uniform.

While tinted lenses theoretically are prescribed primarily to provide protection from the sun, in recent years pastel tints that create a fashion effect have become extremely popular. The best method used to obtain these tints on glass lenses is the coating procedure. Almost any color can be ordered, whereas conventional tints obtained by adding an oxide to the ingredients of clear glass are limited. Manufacturers of color coatings make available kits of sample tints and provide accurate absorption curves, allowing the practitioner to be guided by the patient's needs (one coating company advertises more than 100 varieties).

Most now include antireflection layers on color-coated lenses. This is an excellent advantage since reducing the reflections adds to the attractiveness of the eyewear.

A possible disadvantage of a color-coated lens is the slight metallic look that some patients find objectionable. However, newer processes involved in the coating procedure have considerably reduced this problem.

Coated lenses can be ordered to create special effects. Today, for a fashion look the coating most often requested gives a mirrored finish to the front surface. This mirror coating is usually applied over yellow, gray, brown, or green tints. Lenses can also be coated and/or mirror coated so that either the upper portion is a deeper color than the lower (single gradient density lenses) or the upper and lower parts of the lenses are coated the deep color (double gradient density lenses). Manufacturers claim these special coatings reduce abnormal overhead glare and excessive brightness from "shiny" surfaces such as water, sand, or snow, but they are usually ordered for a fashion effect.

PROTECTIVE LAYERS FOR ANTIREFLECTION AND COLOR COATINGS

At one time, the principle disadvantage of wearing lenses treated with antireflection and color coatings was the difficulty encountered in keeping them clean. They attracted dust and dirt; if the lens was wiped dry or cleaned with silicone papers, abrasive material often marred the coatings.

A durable hard layer that has been developed almost eliminates these problems when it is applied over an antireflection and/or color coating. Lenses thus treated can be cleaned by any conventional method. However, it is still best to wash the lenses whenever possible, for a smear-free surface.

Some laboratories include the protective layer with the antireflection and/or color coating; others supply it only when ordered. It is best to be specific; the advantages offered by the protective layer are such that it should always be included because it also prevents the "peeling off" of the other coatings.

COATINGS FOR PLASTIC LENSES

The major change in the manufacture of CR 39 lenses within the past 5 years is the wide availability of scratch-resistant coatings. While proper cleaning (holding the lenses under running water before wiping clean) keeps surfaces from being marred, practitioners sometimes hesitated to prescribe hard-resin CR 39, which were not as scratch-resistant as glass lenses.

Two processes were made available in the United States at about the same time: Hi-Quartz by Hoya Lens (this scratch-resistant coating was first used in Japan) and Diamond-film by Berg Industries. Originally the coating was available only on the convex surface; in 1979 it became possible to order the coating on both lens surfaces. This was an advantage because the CR 39 lens could now be cleaned like a glass lens. However, both the Hoya and Berg coatings at that time could crack if subjected to high heat. Frame adjustments requiring heat were made with the lenses out of the mountings. Patients reported some lenses "crackled" when worn in hot desert climates.

Today these widely available factory-coated abrasion-resistant CR 39 lenses are generally very satisfactory. The coating is placed by some manufacturers on the outside surface only and by others on both surfaces. There is a complete range in single-vision and multifocal prescriptions.

Sometimes these are identified as "in-mold" coatings. "In-mold" usually means that the lens can be easily tinted to any desired shade (surmounting a problem with the original coatings) and that there will be consistency in color. Blotchy dying/color streaking is eliminated. Color does not build up at the segment dividing lines. Factory applied coatings are so sophisticated that they are usually guaranteed to stay intact for the lifetime of the lens (hard coatings applied by the local laboratory to CR 39 lenses are rarely as satisfactory).

Some of the trade names used by various optical manufacturers include Permalite (American Optical), RLX II (Armorlite), Supremacy Kote (Coburn), SRC (Vision-Ease), Super Shield (Silor), Diacoat II (Seiko), and Perma-Gard (Sola).

The practitioner needs to know that "in-mold" usually means the coating is only on the outside surface of the lens. The local laboratory should be asked for updates, since they occur frequently in this area.

While scratch-resistant coatings are not prescribed primarily as antireflection coatings, they result in an increase in antireflection properties and light transmission. Clear CR 39 uncoated lenses transmit about 93% of incident light, which increases to about 96% when a scratch-resistant coating is applied.

Since the hard coatings are protective, a tinted CR 39 lens cannot be bleached for a different shade or another color (color change is a simple procedure on uncoated CR 39 lenses). Originally there were problems in achieving certain hues in tinted lenses with scratch-resistant layers. (The pink tints appeared to be the least altered.) A solution has been found and all available colors are accurately reproduced. However, there are a few multifocal hard-resin designs that cannot be coated. Query the local laboratory when in doubt.

Scratch-resistant coatings appear to have their greatest value when used on aphakic lenses. The typical cataract patient is elderly and tends to fall asleep while wearing spectacles, which then fall off the face. When the eyewear is not worn, the bulbous outside surface tends to tip and may contact rough surfaces that could scratch unprotected lenses.

While there are advantages in prescribing hard coatings, they are ordered only on about 15% to 20% of the CR 39 lenses dispensed in the United States. Probably the higher cost is a factor because the newer designs are certainly easy to keep scratch free. It usually takes only a little extra care in cleaning (the lenses should be run under water before they are wiped dry).

Note: All polycarbonate plastic lenses have scratch-resistant coatings placed on both surfaces at the factory level. These are discussed in Chapter 7, "Plastic Ophthalmic Lenses."

EDGE COATINGS FOR MINUS LENSES

The local laboratory can apply edge coatings on CR 39 high minus lenses to eliminate the opaqueness of the bevels. The best cosmetic effect is achieved when the coating is a light shade matching a light rimmed frame. Dark shades give a "tunnel" effect to the eyewear (e.g., black plastic frame, black edge coating; deep amber rims, darkish brown-edge lenses). It is always best to show samples of edge coatings to the patient before ordering. They are stark looking and often a better solution is tinting the entire lens a soft hue.

Note: Colored edge coatings are available for glass lenses, but they are rarely used. Glass bevels do not have an opaque look.

Chapter 9

PRESCRIBING ABSORPTIVE LENSES

INTRODUCTION

Absorptive lenses are designed either to prevent certain wavelengths from entering the eye or to reduce the intensity of those wavelengths that do enter. While even in 350 B.C. absorptive lenses were known to help patients with acute needs—such as glassblowers exposed to excessive ultraviolet (UV) and infrared (IR) radiations—the comfort afforded when visible light of high intensities is absorbed has only recently been realized. This understanding is largely the result of research making available lens tints that provide adequate protection for every need. Further enhancement of the role of absorptive lenses has resulted from the involvement of styling experts who consistently promote sunwear as desirable fashion accessories that add interest and intrigue to face and costume.

PROPERTIES OF RADIANT ENERGY

Light is a form of radiant energy, electromagnetic in nature and described by specific wavelengths. The wavelengths of radiant energy extend from the shortest cosmic waves, 10^{-14}m in length, to the longest power-transmission wavelengths at 10^8m. Of these, only the range from 380 to 780nm (where 1 nm = 10^{-9}m) can be perceived by the human eye. This is called the visible spectrum, or "light," where the visual system interprets the individual wavelengths as colors. However, the practitioner is concerned not only with the visible spectrum, but also with the wavelengths extending slightly to each side.

The ultraviolet (UV) rays are in the continuation of the visible spectrum at the blue end and consist of UVA from 315 to 400 nm, UVB from 280 to 315nm, and UVC from 100 to 280nm. The infrared (IR) radiations are off the red end of the visible spectrum and are described as the near IR from 700 to 1400nm, the intermediate IR from 1400 to 5000nm, and the far IR from 5000 to 1,000,000nm. Overexposure to these rays can result in ocular discomfort and pathological involvement of the eye and its adnexa.

UVA and UVB rays are found in sunlight; the UVC is filtered from sunlight by the earth's atmosphere, especially the ozone layer. Human overexposure to UV is most likely at high altitudes, where the atmosphere is thin, and in the sunlight reflected from any shimmery area like snow or water. Overexposure is also possible from man-made sources, such as the arcs created during electric welding, and the ultraviolet lamps used for a variety of purposes from germicidal applications to pleasurable tanning. Prolonged overexposure to UV rays can result in inflammation of the cornea and the conjunctiva, cancers of the eye and its adnexa, cataracts, pterygia, and retinal disease, to name a few of the implicated disorders.

IR rays can be hazardous, too. Looking directly at sources that produce these radiations—direct sunlight, molten substances such as glass and metal, arc lamps, and infrared lamps—can result in clouding of the crystalline lens and/or lesions of the retina and choroid if the radiations are of sufficient intensity and duration.

Exposure to the visible spectrum, 380 to 760nm, does not normally lead to pathological disorders. However, individuals who are extremely sensitive to light rays found in normal illumination may experience symptoms described as eyestrain and eye fatigue, and overexposure to the short wavelength (blue) part of the visible spectrum is suspected to contribute to certain retinal dysfunctions.

CLASSIFICATION OF CONVENTIONAL TINTS FOR GLASS LENSES

Clear crown glass lenses transmit 90% to 92% of the radiation between 300 to 4000nm. These lenses absorb almost 100% of the radiations below 300nm, the short ultraviolet (UV) rays. Since these absorptions are not always suitable for a specific application, major U.S. manufacturers produce a variety of tinted glass lenses to meet every visual need. Certain chemicals are added in the ingredients of clear glass during the manufacturing process to result in both a color change and transmission characteristics. The color of the lens, however, does not necessarily indicate its absorptive properties. Two pink lenses, appearing the same shade, for instance, may have different transmission curves. The lens color depends on its absorptive value for the visible spectrum only and even then only determines its general effect upon the light rays. A lens, for example, that absorbs the red, green, and yellow wavelengths more than the blue, will appear blue in color.

The addition of cerium oxide also makes a lens more opaque to UV radiation; if ferrous oxide is added, the lens is more opaque to infrared.

Conventional tinted glass lenses are distributed under various trade names, but they can be grouped into one of the following four classifications. The lightest tint in any group is designated by the lowest number or by the letter closest to the beginning of the alphabet.

1. **Lenses that evenly reduce the transmission of the visible spectrum while absorbing UV and IR rays.** These lenses can be light enough for indoor wear or dark enough to be classified as sunlenses. The lighter shades are pink in color and generally designed to transmit 80 to 88% of the visible spectrum. They are recommended to patients who complain of indoor glare. These individuals usually have light skin and/or large pupils, or they may have a psychological need for such a tint. The deeper pinks can be prescribed to albinos for indoor wear (lack of pigment makes these individuals extremely sensitive to light). Pink is also a popular hue and is frequently worn in various tones for its fashion effect.

    Some trade names for glass pink tints are as follows:

MANUFACTURER	TRADE NAME
Bausch & Lomb	Softlite (discontinued)
Shuron-Textron	Tonetex
Titmus Optical	Velvetlite
Vision-Ease	Pink 1
	Pink 2
	Pink 3

    Note: Bausch & Lomb has discontinued production of prescription lenses, but Softlite is such a recognizable name that it is used to identify some plastic pink tints.

The suntints in this category are gray in color and offer the finest protection because they absorb harmful UV and IR radiation without distorting the visible spectrum. These lenses are distributed under the following trade names:

MANUFACTURER	TRADE NAME
Bausch & Lomb	Rayban G31 (medium gray, light transmission 31%)
	Rayban G15 (dark gray, light transmission 15%)
American Optical Corp.	True-color C (medium gray)
	True-color (dark gray)
Vision-Ease	Gray 1
	Gray 2
	Gray 3
Shuron-Textron	Nutrex 1 (light gray)
	Nutrex 2 (medium gray)
	Nutrex 3 (dark gray)
Titmus Optical Co.	TO 30 (medium gray, light transmission 30%)
	TO 20 (dark gray, light transmission 20%)

Note: Bausch & Lomb continues to manufacture Rayban G31 and G15 in plano lenses. They are the best-selling sunlenses in the world.

The choice of a medium-gray or dark-gray tint depends on the patient's subjective reaction to bright illumination. Most prefer the look of the medium color, but if symptoms are acute, it is best to prescribe the deeper shade.

2. **Lens tints that absorb UV radiation, and transmit the visible spectrum evenly.** The pink tints in this category are satisfactory for patients needing an overall reduction of light transmission. These people often complain about general glare. They tend to be light complexioned, and have light eyes and/or large pupils.

Probably the most widely prescribed pink tint was the Cruxite AX (visible light transmission about 83%), distributed by American Optical Corp. Glass lenses in this category are rarely used today, but the name Cruxite remains as identification for some pink-tinted plastic lenses.

The deep shade in this category is Cosmetan, a brown color created by American Optical Corp. The color is available from other manufacturers, for example, Vision-Ease makes brownish shades identified as Tan 1, Tan 2, and Tan 3, which are similar to Cosmetan. While promoted as sunlenses, they are usually prescribed to patients desiring the brown tones for fashion value.

3. **Lenses that absorb UV and IR rays but show some selectivity for the visible spectrum.** The general-purpose lens most used in this category is manufactured by Therminon Lens Co. and distributed with the trade name Therminon; Vision-Ease makes the lens under the name Unisol.

Pale greenish-blue in appearance, it is designated for patients needing a slight reduction in the amount of light that enters the eye. However, unless there is a specific reason for its use, the pink tints which have the same reduction in transmission and do not show selectivity in the visible spectrum, are a better choice. In addition, many patients find the "coke bottle" look of the lens a cosmetic detraction.

The suntints in this category are green in appearance. They are selective in their transmission of the visible spectrum and alter color values slightly. The gray tints are almost always preferable for sunglasses because they absorb harmful radiations without affecting the visible spectrum. However, green is returning as a popular fashion color. Green tints are manufactured under the following trade names:

MANUFACTURER	TRADE NAME
Bausch & Lomb	Rayban 1 (discontinued)
	Rayban 2
	Rayban 3
American Optical Corp.	Calobar B
	Calobar C
	Calobar D
Vision-Ease	Green 1
	Green 2
	Green 3
Titmus Optical Co.	Contra-glare A
	Contra-glare B
	Contra-glare C
	Contra-glare D (very dark)

MANUFACTURER	TRADE NAME
Shuron-Textron	Greentex 1
	Greentex 2
	Greentex 3

Note: Bausch & Lomb continues production of the Rayban 2 and Rayban 3 in plano form because of their popularity in fashion eyewear.

4. **Tints designed for special uses.**   The lenses in this category are highly selective in their absorptive properties. Since each tint is drastically different from any other, they are classified according to color with an explanation of their use.

Yellow-tinted Lenses.   Often referred to as "shooting" lenses, these tints absorb most of the UV rays but have a high transmission for IR. They transmit the visible spectrum by about 70%. Theoretically, the tint "cuts" through early-morning haze to render distant objects more visible. However, studies often concluded this claim was not valid. Scored marksmanship tests, taken with individuals wearing the yellow lenses and compared with scores when the lenses were not worn, showed that the majority were not better marksmen using yellow tinted lens. However, this is a controversial subject. Patients often comment that wearing "shooting glasses" during cloudy/foggy hours improves their marksmanship and others claim the glasses make skiing easier during the twilight hours. This reaction is a definite possibility because the yellow lens has the ability to filter blue light, the shortest wavelength light in the spectrum. The blue can focus in front of the retina resulting in a blurred image on the retina.

American Optical distributes yellow glass lenses under the trade name Hazemaster; Bausch & Lomb identifies them as Kalichrome (available in plano only).

Note: Yellow lenses have become extremely popular as fashion shades and are manufactured by a great number of optical companies in plano form mounted into stylish frames.

At one time, these tints were identified with "television glasses." Theoretically there was increased contrast when viewing a black and white screen. However, studies proved this to be an unscientific fact which was used as an advertising promotion.

Extra-dark Green Lenses.   Visibility is considerably reduced when these lenses are worn since light transmission is a very low 5% to 10%. Distributed under the trade name Noviweld by American Optical Corp. (Bausch & Lomb used the term Industrial Green), their use is restricted to specific industrial wear. Very few manufacturers make this color available.

Dark Smoke Lenses. These lenses were grayish-black in appearance. Since they reduced visibility markedly, they were used only for temporary relief of acute photophobia resulting from a pathological condition. In professional offices throughout the United States, dark smoked-glass lenses have been replaced by "throw-away" cardboard-framed plastic designs as a precaution against transmitting eye infections.

GLASS LENSES EMPLOYING IMBEDDED CHEMICAL SUBSTANCES FOR THEIR ABSORPTIVE PROPERTIES

Polaroid Lenses. The polarized lens is designed to eliminate glare reflected from flat surfaces at certain angles. Prescription polaroids are fashioned from films of polarizing material laminated between clear or lightly tinted glass lenses or plastic lenses. The polarizing material consists of nitrocellulose packed with ultramicroscopic crystals of herepathite having their optic axes parallel to one another. Most polarized filters transmit about 37% of incident light. Quality polaroid sunlenses function in an excellent manner to reduce glare from "shiny" horizontal surfaces, such as highways, water, or snow.

For many years Polaroid lenses were available exclusively through American Optical Corp. Later a polarized lens was distributed by Liberty Optical Co. under the trade name Vergopol. At present almost all quality Polaroid prescription lenses are manufactured in Japan and distributed in the United States by Melibrand under the trade name Polar-ray. In single-vision lenses they are available in a number of very attractive colors as well as the conventional gray C (deep gray) sunshade. The gray C and a medium gray are also made in a straight-top D-style 25mm bifocal and a straight-top 7 × 25mm trifocal. Oversize glass lenses are easily available in single-vision designs, but size limitations in the multifocal styles should be checked with the local laboratory. Since the manufacturing process is relatively complicated, the cost of prescription polaroids is higher than prescription lenses of conventional tints.

Photochromic (Sunsensor) Lenses. Photochromics, promoted to the public as light-sensitive sunsensor lenses and once called photochromatic lenses, are designed to darken when exposed to UV radiation. The color change is achieved by the addition of silver halide crystals evenly dispersed in the glass. Each is about 1/100,000mm in diameter, tightly packed so as to avoid scattering of visible light.

There are a number of photochromic designs widely advertised to the profession and to the public. Most are manufactured by Corning Glass Works and sold to optical companies, each of whom then distributes them under an individual label. Before discussing the characteristics of each design, there are fundamentals applicable to all that need to be understood.

1. Photochromic lenses darken only when exposed to ultra-violet rays. If these radiations are blocked (for instance, behind the windshield of a car), the lenses remain in the lightened stage. Conversely, the lenses may darken on a dull day when UV rays are in the atmosphere or indoors under UV lights.

2. Photochromic lenses need to go through as many as ten light-to-dark cycles before they will darken to potential.

3. If photochromic lenses are not worn for a period of time, usually exceeding a month, the light-to-dark cycles have to be repeated. The darkening performance never deteriorates, however, and can be reactivated indefinitely.

4. Photochromic lenses may darken but not to their maximum on a foggy or misty day.

5. The color change in photochromic lenses is affected by the temperature; the colder the day, the darker they will become. Some, like Bausch & Lomb's Ambermatic, reach a different maximum color on cold days.

6. The prescription must be close to the same for both eyes. If the right lens, for instance, is +3.00 −1.00 × 90 and the left a +6.00D sphere, the lenses will not darken evenly.

7. Photochromic lenses are usually thicker than conventional lenses. While density is 2.54g/ml and index is 1.523, the same as standard crown glass, additional weight theoretically, should not be a problem. However, the thicker the lens the darker it will get for a given sunlight exposure, so local laboratories insist upon determining the thickness.

8. The color change in photochromic lenses may be altered in an unpredictable fashion if lens coatings are used. The lens may stay in a darkened stage when the patient returns indoors or may darken to a color foreign to the design.

9. All the photochromics of a specific model do not lighten and darken in an absolute pattern. Batches produced one month can and will vary from those manufactured at a later date. Photochromic lenses should therefore be ordered in pairs.

10. While photochromic designs absorb UV radiations, they all transmit IR. If a patient is exposed excessively or continuously to direct or reflected sunlight, molten glass/molten metal glass lenses such as Bausch & Lomb's Rayban G15 and G31, which absorb IR as well as UV rays, need to be prescribed.

11. Photochromic lenses should be chemically tempered to make them impact-resistant. Heat treating lowers the transmission and, as with all lenses processed in the latter manner, makes them more susceptible to spontaneous breakage (see Chapter 10, "Impact-Resistant [Safety] Lenses").

Specific Photochromic Designs

Note: The percent of transmission given varies slightly depending on lens thickness, temperature, and tempering state. Transmission curves are determined by lens exposure to natural sunlight at 25°C (77°F). The lenses are tested in plano form, 2mm thick.

1. Photogray Lenses. The first photochromic lenses were introduced in 1968; they are still prescribed. In the palest stage light transmission is 83%, making them ideal indoor lenses. When darkened to their maximum, the 44% transmission results in a medium gray outdoor tint comfortable for most patients. Photograys were available in a one-piece Ultex A-style bifocal and in Executive bifocals and trifocals, but they had the inherent problems characteristic of these designs. The Executive with its prominent "shelflike" segment lines and necessary thickness is cosmetically unattractive. The Ultex "half-moon" with its optical center 19mm below the segment division resulted in considerable image jump.

2. Photosun Lenses. The next photochromics to be introduced were Photosun lenses. The Photosun designs are light gray indoors with 65% light transmission. In the maximum darkness stage, the lens becomes a dark gray having 20% light transmission. It is too dark for comfortable indoor vision and is unsafe for night driving. They were manufactured in Executive-style and Ultex "half-moon" bifocals. Because of the absorption characteristics, the lens had limited use and was soon discontinued. A Photosun II is now manufactured and discussed later in this chapter.

3. Photobrown Lenses.   These lenses became available in 1974. Promoted as clear indoors with an average light transmission of 88%, there was a pale residual yellowish-green tint that was not attractive. Maximum darkness was advertised as 45% light transmission, but research showed the average darkest stage to be 59%. The lenses did not darken sufficiently in bright sunlight and the design was discontinued. Soon a dark Photobrown was introduced. The dark Photobrown had about 64% transmission indoors, too dark for proper visual efficiency. The maximum 22% sunlight exposure made this an efficient out-of-doors color for patients desiring a deep tint. Availability in multifocals was markedly limited and very few of these lenses were prescribed.

4. Fused Light and Dark Photochromics.   These designs in 1975 were a welcome addition for the presbyopic patient. Easily available in an ST25mm bifocal and an ST7/25mm trifocal, other fused designs could be factory ordered. In all cases, however, the segments are clear, fused onto a photochromic major blank so the reading area stays lighter in the darkening stage. The fused light was very popular, a light yellowish-tan in the lightest 88% transmission stage and becoming a comfortable 38% when exposed to bright sunlight. In the darkened stage, the lens was slightly deeper in color than a gray #2 tint. The fused dark was not requested often, having 66% light transmission indoors and 16% (a dark gray color) out-of-doors. Today the prescribed fused multifocals are the Photogray Extra designs.

5. Photogray Extra™.   This is currently the most popular photochromic lens and distributed by all major glass manufacturers. In its lightest stage, the tint at 85% transmission is comparable to a Photogray design. At its darkest stage, which is achieved in bright sunshine, the color becomes a deep gray with 22% transmission. The change from light to dark takes place in about 60 seconds, which is quicker than previous photochromics. Photogray Extra is available in single-vision, executive bifocals and all popular-size fused, straight-top multifocals (ST25mm, ST28mm, ST35mm bifocals; ST7–25; ST7–28mm trifocals and double-segment occupational designs, depending upon specific manufacturer/ distributor). The segment glass is clear, so the near/intermediate areas remain in a lighter shade when the lens darkens. Photogray Extra lenses are also manufactured in one-piece, seamless/blended bifocals and progressive-addition designs.

6. Photobrown Extra.   This lens is a deep brown color in the darkest stage, with 25% light transmission. In the faded stage, it has 86% transmission. The design is not widely prescribed, so it is best to query the local laboratory for current availability of multifocal styles. In the fused designs, the segment areas are lighter than the distance when the lens is exposed to bright illumination.

7. *Photosun II.*   Photosun II is a recently introduced photochromic designed for use as a sun lens in both the faded and darkened stages. The lens is a gray color and when lightened becomes a medium gray with 40% light transmission. In the darkest stage it transmits 12% of the visible light. On hot days the lenses reveal a subdued deep gray. The reaction to temperature changes is obvious.

The Photosun II is not for the patient having only one pair of glasses. The color in the faded stage is too dark indoors and dangerous for night driving. Many patients find it too deep for comfort in the darkest stage, and it may adversely affect visual acuity. Only a few multifocal designs are available, so the laboratory needs to be queried for availability.

8. *Photogray II.*   The Photogray II (Figure 9.1) has a significantly faster darkening/fading cycle than the original Photogray. Within 5 minutes it regains 70% of its clearness when the patient returns indoors. In its lightest form there is 87% transmission with a maximum darkness of 42% transmission. With the introduction of Photogray II, it is likely the original Photogray may not be available.

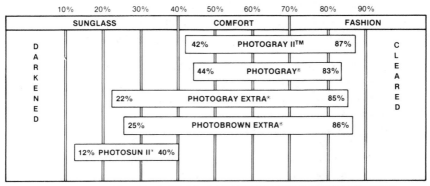

FIGURE 9.1   *Photogray II*

9. Sun Magic Photochromics. These lenses are manufactured by Scholt Optical Glass and differ from other photochromics in that less time is needed for the fading stage after darkening has taken place. They are useful for patients needing "instant" clearer lenses when returning to an indoor environment. They are available only in plano and single vision corrections in a wide variety of colors that include gray, brown, tan, green, and blue.

10. Custom Photochromic Lenses. Corning can produce any color with the desired absorption curves and makes specific lenses available as exclusives to optical companies upon request. The lenses can be solid or gradient colors.

Bausch & Lomb, for example, distributes Rayban Ambermatic lenses with unique optical and physical characteristics. In its lightest stage the lens has 65% transmission and becomes a yellow-amber designed to cut through haze on a cloudy day. Maximum darkness results in a lens having 20% light transmission. In the dark form the Rayban Ambermatic differs in color because of a dramatic response to temperature. On warm days the lens is a brown shade; on a marginally bright, warm day the color may be a light brown. On cold, sunny days the tone is a deep gray, slightly lighter like Rayban G15.

Corning has made exclusive pink and blue photochromics for Hoya Lens. Obviously, they have limited use but are attractive as fashion shades.

11. Corning Photochromic Filter Lenses. The Corning Photochromic Filter (CPF) series are lenses distributed by Corning Medical Optics for wear by low-vision patients. Three designs were originally released: CPF 511, CPF 527, and CPF 550. These lenses absorb UV radiation as well as the blue end of the visible spectrum. The three digits refer to the wavelength in nanometers to which the lenses attenuate.

CPF lenses have a very distinctive color range. Depending on the design, they vary from red to yellow-amber. Like all photochromics, the lenses fade in low illumination and darken in bright sunlight. Specifically designed to cut acute glare that adversely affects the partially sighted, CPF lenses are considered a major breakthrough, since certain pathologies result in a glare factor that limits visibility.

The CPF 511 lens has 16% light transmission in the darkened stage, with resultant deep orange-yellow color. The lightened stage is a yellow-amber tone exhibiting 47% transmission. The CPF 511 is recommended for patients with immature cataracts, diabetic retinopathy, and those who are aphakes.

CPF 527 has 12% transmission in the darkest stage and 37% in the lightest. Both stages are deep tones, with the lighter being an orange-amber color. CPF 527 is recommended for patients with severe photophobia regardless of cause.

The CPF 550 is a very dark lens, 5% transmission in the darkened stage (seriously affecting the vision of a normally sighted person), becoming a reddish-amber in the lightened stage, with 21% transmission. CPF 550 lenses are designed for patients with retinitis pigmentosa.

Before prescribing the CPF series, the literature prepared by Corning Medical Optics should be studied carefully; each lens has transmission properties making it best (or suitable) for patients with certain vision problems and/or pathological conditions.

CPF lenses are available in plano form as well as prescription single-vision, bifocal, trifocal, and lenticular designs. Only certain optical laboratories can finish the prescription lenses, so inquiry about ordering procedures is critical. Information regarding the CPF series is available by contacting: Corning Glass Works, Optical Products Department, Corning, NY 14831.

PHOTOLITE PLASTIC PHOTOCHROMICS

Photolites are plastic photochromic lenses manufactured by American Optical Corp., designed primarily as fashion tints. They do not darken sufficiently for use as sunlenses. The 90% to 92% indoor transmission is comparable to that of a clear lens. In bright sunlight Photolites become light blue in color.

Unlike glass photochromics that make use of silver halides, the color change in Photolites works through an organic compound applied to the lens surface. Unfortunately, the blue color fades after prolonged exposure to UV radiations, thus limiting UV absorption. They are manufactured in single vision only and are not widely prescribed.

Note: As of this writing, there are plastic photochromic lenses advertised as having the capacity to darken like glass photochromics. They are too new to judge.

HARD-RESIN CR 39 (PLASTIC) ABSORPTIVE LENSES

Tints in any desired shade are easily obtained by dyeing a plastic CR39 lens. The most popular fashion hues appear to be soft pinks and blues, dove gray, pale tan, and some shades of green and yellow. If light transmission is 80% to 85%, these colors do not abnormally distort the visible spectrum.

Absorptive curves for plastic lenses are rarely if ever made available, but if the fashion shades are vivid, natural colors will appear distorted or drastically altered. Patients must be discouraged from wearing such deep tones when driving a car, operating a motorcycle, or flying a plane, because the change in color perception could result in a misinterpretation of important signals (e.g., red and green lights). These tints are especially dangerous if worn at night and/or in combination with tinted windshields.

Initially, the use of hard coatings to make the surfaces of CR 39 lenses scratch resistant resulted in an inability to tint such lenses properly. For the most part these problems have been solved.

There are now available CR 39 polarized bifocals in a 22mm round design. The standard shades are Gray A and Gray C tints, but these hard-resin lenses can be dyed to achieve a wider range of colors. There may be additions in color and bifocal style, so it is best to query the local laboratory for availability.

Polar-lite is a polarized lens recently appearing on the U.S. market. Manufactured in Japan, it is a molded CR 39 lens. Instead of being laminated, the polarizing material is in the lens itself. By eliminating the lamination, possible splitting of the filter from the lens is impossible. The lens is also lighter in weight than laminated designs. Polar-lite is available in several colors in single vision and in a flat-top 28mm bifocal, Gray A only. This is a rather pale hue, but since the material is CR 39, the lens can be tinted a deeper shade. It is expected that additional standard colors will be available soon.

Literature suggests that Polar-lite can be coated for a mirrored effect, but practitioners should approach this procedure with caution. Mirror coatings tend not to stay intact when applied to plastic lenses, but it is hoped that this problem will soon be solved.

Absorption curves for UV and IR radiations, as well as the visible spectrum, vary according to individual Polaroid designs. Manufacturers should be queried for specifics.

Younger Optics makes four special CR 39 plastic lenses designed to reduce some of the symptoms associated with specific eye disorders (however, the manufacturer does not claim therapeutic effects). The lenses are called the Younger Protective Lens Series: PLS 400, PLS 530, PLS 540, and PLS 550. They virtually cut off all UV and visible blue light below the wavelengths designated by the product number. The PLS 400 designs are almost clear but have a golden cast, the PLS 530 lenses are orange-amber in color, the PLS 540 are brown, and the PLS 550 lenses are reddish. Some of Younger Optics' recommendations are:

> PLS 400 Lenses
> For those taking photosensitizing medications; for patients with pterygiums or pingueculae.

PLS 530 Lenses
For patients with developing cataracts, extreme light
sensitivity (albinism), corneal dystrophy, and diabetic
retinopathy.

PLS 540
Basically a sunlens for contact lens wearers, skiers,
boaters, and mountain climbers.

PLS 550 Lenses
For pathological conditions; macular degeneration, glau-
coma, and retinitis pigmentosa.

The determination of lens recommendation is made by the eye-care
professional who can query the local laboratory for additional literature.
The Younger Protective Lens Series is available in a wide range of bifocal
styles including flat-top 25mm, 28mm, and 35mm; round 22mm and
40mm; seamless designs; and progressive addition lenses. Since the lenses
are CR 39, color can be added by conventional tinting methods without
changing the basic UV protective properties.

POLYCARBONATE PLASTIC ABSORPTIVE LENSES

All polycarbonate lenses absorb the harmful UV radiation. The addition
of color creates a fashion look and/or gives tints for use out-of-doors.
Polycarbonate lenses have hard coatings on both surfaces, so obtaining
deep shades for sunwear has been a problem. However, this should be
solved in the near future.

COLOR COATINGS FOR GLASS LENSES

Absorptive curves for color coatings applied to glass lenses are usually
available from the manufacturer. Some absorb IR as well as UV rays.
In most cases the practitioner can prescribe them knowing their effects
on the various wavelengths. The lens coatings that are vivid in color for
a fashion effect have the same dangers as the bright plastic tints. The
hues that are very, very pale and appear to be just a "cast" of color
have a light transmission of about 88 to 90% and are as safe to wear as
clear lenses.

EFFECT OF PRESCRIPTION ON LENS COLOR

Color is uniform in a conventional tinted glass lens (an oxide is added
to the ingredients of clear glass) only when center and edge thicknesses
are equal (plano). When tinted prescription lenses are deep in intensity,

the problem of maintaining uniform color can be critical.

A convex lens, being thicker in the center, has a deeper color in that area. With a concave correction, the reverse is true; the center, which is thinner than the edges, will be a lighter shade. A cylindrical correction can appear to have a darker or lighter band of color, depending on the prescription.

When the correction involved is less than ±2.00D, the difference in color is not obvious enough to present a problem. In a lens correction ±2.25D to ±4.00D, usually the color differences can be minimized effectively by requesting the laboratory to control thickness (i.e., to keep the center of minus lenses thicker than conventional lenses). A frame can be dispensed that limits the horizontal box measurement of the lens to 50mm to 52mm. The larger the lens, the more obvious the color variation.

When the correction is greater than ±4.00D, or if it varies greatly between the two eyes (e.g., +1.00D for the right eye and –3.00D for the left eye), it is always necessary to use some method of tinting that results in uniform color. There are three possibilities: One involves the use of plastic lenses; another, coating the lens the desired tint; the third uses glass uniform-density laminated lenses.

The tint of a plastic lens is impregnated into the lens surface, making it uniform regardless of the correction. However, several precautions are necessary when prescribing plastic sunlenses. While they satisfactorily cut down general illumination and eliminate harmful UV rays, they do not absorb IR light. If the patient is exposed continuously to IR radiation (e.g., a glassblower or an outdoor worker in the desert), it is necessary to prescribe a lens having known absorptive properties.

Note: Several lens manufacturers advertise an IF-absorbing prescription plastic design, but studies need to be done to verify the claims.

Care of plastic CR39 lenses is more involved than those fashioned of glass, and this may be an inconvenience when sunglasses are involved. To maintain a scratch-free surface, dust must be washed off the lens before wiping clean. Silicone papers cannot be used, because they mar the lenses. On the other hand, the added safety of plastic lenses is often an important consideration, particularly when worn while operating a motor vehicle.

Note: If the lens surface has a scratch-resistant coating, it can be cleaned by any conventional method. However, most CR 39 lenses manufactured in this manner have the coating only on the front surface.

Uniform color can also be obtained by applying a color coating to a clear glass lens. The lens is cut to the required size and shape before the coating process takes place. This makes it possible to prescribe large sunlenses that offer maximum protection. Absorption curves of color coatings are available, allowing the practitioner to prescribe them when absorption properties are critical to the patient's needs.

There are a few disadvantages that need to be considered when prescribing color-coated glass lenses. The coating has a "metallic" look, although this problem is greatly lessened when the color is applied by a quality laboratory. Another disadvantage may be that coated lenses need to be cleaned frequently. They attract dust that adheres to the lens surface. To be cleaned properly, they should be run under warm water before wiping clean. The problem is minimized with a permanent clear coating designed to allow silicone papers to be used on coated lenses.

Prescribing a uniform-density laminated glass lens is another method of controlling color in a prescription lens. To achieve the desired results a tinted plano lens is laminated to the prescription clear lens. These lenses are rarely used in the United States. They are difficult to manufacture in a finished size greater than a 48mm horizontal box measurement, making them too small for most sunwear fashions. The method of manufacture results in a relatively heavy lens, and when high corrections are involved, these lenses are highly impractical. In addition, the laminated layers have a tendency to separate.

AVAILABILITY OF TINTED LENS PRESCRIPTIONS

A drastic change has taken place in the manufacture and stocking of glass absorptive lenses. Tinted hard-resin lenses are prescribed with increasing frequency and are colored at the local laboratory. For this reason, glass lenses that have an oxide added in the manufacturing process are no longer readily available in various powers and a wide selection of colors. It is rare for a local laboratory to maintain a prescription inventory of glass single-vision tinted lenses in shades other than light pink, medium gray, and dark gray. Major manufacturers of conventional bifocals and trifocals make them, in addition to the clear form, in a soft pink and a gray suntint, but rarely in other shades. Although this may appear as a limitation in availability, it should be remembered that a clear glass lens can be color coated to any desired tone. Every coating company distributes kits featuring sample colors that can be easily duplicated. Some are gradient for a fashion effect. Photochromic lenses are usually stocked at the local laboratory in Photogray Extra in a complete range of prescriptions and multifocal designs. However, other kinds of photochromic lenses are often available within a short waiting period.

SUNFRAME FASHIONS

Tinted plano lenses in currently popular fashion colors and suntints are readily obtained from local laboratories. They are available in an uncut form, but most practitioners order them already mounted in fashionable sunframes. UV absorbers are found in all quality lenses. There are planos in CR 39 that also absorb IR radiations.

Almost every major frame manufacturer introduces a new line of sunfashions twice a year and sometimes as often as four times a year. These designs create a specific type of fashion value that is rarely achieved when a conventional frame is dispensed for sunwear. Absorptive properties of the lenses must be ascertained so that the practitioner can properly recommend them for specific needs.

When dark lenses are mounted into a plastic frame that is not designed for sunglasses, the patient is often justifiably disappointed in the cosmetic effect. They can look "too small," an illusion resulting from the darkness of the lenses contrasting with skin tone, although this effect is becoming popular with young wearers.

Sunglasses that curve toward the temples (goggle sunframes) are sometimes worn by skiers and contact lens patients. When objects are viewed through the periphery of a lens mounted into a "curved" frame, distortion is present. Patients may find this extremely annoying even if the distortion is slight. When a high prescription is involved, the problem can be critical. The higher the correction, the greater is the cylindrical effect that results in distortion (see Chapter 14, "Prescription Changes Induced by Lens Tilt"). It is usually best not to recommend a "goggle" curved-frame design for any prescription lens. However, in corrections up to ±1.00D the distortion may be slight enough that patients can tolerate it, particularly if the angle of the curvature is limited to 10°.

Fit-over frames utilizing tinted plano lenses are cumbersome, make a poor appearance, and can mar the surface of the prescription lenses. All corrections are available in suntints; surprisingly, patients may not be aware of this, particularly those who need high-power lenses.

WHEN TO PRESCRIBE SUNWEAR

All patients benefit from wearing quality tinted lenses (in prescription if necessary) when sunlight is bright or the glare excessive. These tints provide a more comfortable environment and improve visual acuity adversely affected by annoying reflections. For some patients, sunwear is a necessity. Wearers of hard contact lenses, for instance, are rarely comfortable out-of-doors without adequate protection against the sun's rays.

The gray glass tints that absorb the UV and IR radiation without altering the visible spectrum offer the finest complete sunwear protection. The shade prescribed depends upon subjective symptoms. If the patient reports mild annoyance in bright illumination, the medium gray tint is usually the best choice.

Since in actuality most patients need only UV-absorbing lenses, quality CR 39, polycarbonates, and photochromic designs offer proper protection. In addition, plano plastic lenses are now easily available with IR absorbers, although the selection of frame styles is limited.

When patients request a special tint for its fashion value, the practitioner needs to exercise professional judgment, since deeply hued fashion colors drastically alter the visible spectrum.

Chapter 10

IMPACT-RESISTANT (SAFETY) LENSES

INTRODUCTION

A policy statement issued by the federal Food and Drug Administration (FDA) made it illegal not to prescribe impact-resistant lenses as of January 1, 1972. If the practitioner decides for a specific case not to prescribe them, certain conditions need to be followed. These are stated under section (c) of the law and are quoted in this chapter.

The essentials of the law—those factors particularly pertinent to the practitioner—are noted in this introduction. However, changes are possible and it is the practitioner's responsibility to know the legal aspects affecting the eye-care professions. Any additional information desired may be obtained by querying the federal government. Local laboratories also can be queried, because they are knowledgeable about all changes. As of January 1, 1972, the following ruling regarding impact-resistant lenses became law:

Title 21—Food and Drugs

Chapter 1—Food and Drug Administration
Department of Health, Education, and Welfare
Subchapter A—General

Part 3—statements of general policy or interpretation
Use of Impact-Resistant lenses in Eyeglasses and Sunglasses. . . .

(a) Examination of data available on the frequency of eye injuries resulting from the shattering of ordinary crown glass lenses
indicate that the use of such lenses constitutes an avoidable hazard
to the eye of the wearer.

(b) The consensus of the ophthalmic community is that the
number of eye injuries would be substantially reduced by the
use in eyeglasses and sunglasses of either plastic lenses, heat-
treated crown glass lenses, or lenses made impact-resistant by
other methods.

(c) To protect the public more adequately from potential eye
injury, eyeglasses and sunglasses must be fitted with impact-resistant lenses, except in those cases where the physician or optometrist finds that such lenses will not fulfill the visual requirements
of the particular patient, directs in writing the use of other lenses,
and gives written notification thereof to the patient.

(d) The physician or optometrist shall have the option of ordering heat-treated glass lenses, plastic lenses, laminated glass lenses,
or glass lenses made impact-resistant by other methods; however,
all such lenses must be capable of withstanding an impact test
in which a ⅝ inch steel ball weighing approximately 0.56 ounce
is dropped from a height of 50 inches upon the horizontal upper
surface of the lens. . . .

Lenses classified as impact-resistant and often referred .to as safety
lenses have been available for many years. However, until the above
policy statement by the FDA made it illegal not to prescribe impact-
resistant lenses, they were recommended at the discretion of the practitioner. Now when prescribing non-impact-resistant lenses, certain conditions must be followed; they are stated under section (c). As a result,
almost all lenses used in the United States are manufactured of an impact-
resistant material or are made impact-resistant by certain methods that
give them a protective quality. Few eye-care professionals ever apply
the exception stated under (c), since it makes them more susceptible to
possible legal complications.

The law includes a complete explanation of the method that must be
used to test lenses (e.g., where the ball will strike the lens). These
specifications are followed by the laboratory that fills the prescription.
If the practitioner tempers lenses in the office, detailed information regarding the equipment and related matters can be obtained by querying
the federal government.

Until the law became effective, the term "safety lenses" was used
synonymously with "impact-resistant lenses." However, patient confu-

sion—most lay persons interpret "safety" as meaning an unbreakable lens—has resulted in a recommendation by the American Optometric Association that the term "safety lenses" be eliminated. Instead, an explanation should be offered the patient that although impact-resistant lenses are designed to withstand considerable pressure, any lens can and will break if struck with enough force (the possible exception being polycarbonate lenses).

TYPES OF IMPACT-RESISTANT LENSES

Lenses classified as impact-resistant are available in a number of forms. The best are manufactured from a hard-resin material, CR 39 plastic, and polycarbonate lenses. Others are made of optical-quality glass modified to give a protective quality. Impact-resistant lenses made of glass are further subdivided into chemically tempered, heat-treated (sometimes called "air-treated"), and laminated lenses.

Polycarbonate Lenses and Plastic (Hard-resin CR 39) Lenses

There are many ramifications involving plastic lenses, particularly the tremendous strides made in the design of both single-vision and multifocal lenses. Chapter 7, "Plastic Ophthalmic Lenses" is devoted exclusively to this subject. This chapter concerns itself with the advantages from a safety viewpoint.

Polycarbonate lenses are advertised as virtually unbreakable. The same material is used in the manufacture of bullet-proof vests. These designs offer the patient the most protection from potential injury.

CR 39 lenses exhibit a high degree of safety. Research shows that a chemically tempered lens appears to withstand the same force as a plastic CR 39, although when it does break, there is a kickback property whereby glass particles can be imbedded into the eye tissue and surrounding facial area. These bits of glass are often difficult to locate and remove, particularly if a clear (transparent) lens breaks. This kickback property was not noted when hard-resin lenses were broken during scientific studies; the pieces there were likely to be large rather than splinters and tended to stay contained in the frame.

Glass Impact-resistant Lenses

Chemically Tempered Lenses.   Chemical strengthening is the best process used to make conventional glass lenses impact resistant. It was developed for ophthalmic use by Corning Glass Works when it became obvious that the FDA ruling might force practitioners to prescribe heat-treated (air-tempered) lenses, which have serious drawbacks as discussed later in this chapter. Chemical tempering involves a chemical ion exchange between sodium ions in the glass and potassium ions in a specially prepared salt bath. Although introduced about 2 decades ago, its use had been limited primarily to automobile and aircraft windshields and to laboratory glassware.

There are several advantages to prescribing chemically tempered over heat-treated lenses. Chemically tempered lenses maintain excellent optics without the warpage noted on the surfaces of air-tempered lenses. It is possible to manufacture a chemically tempered lens in a thinner form and still comply with the FDA ruling. Chemically treated lenses in the 1.3- to 1.5mm minimum thickness range have proven under testing conditions to be stronger than 2.2mm heat-treated lenses.

The chemical strengthening process takes longer than heat treating. The lenses are placed for 15 to 16 hours in the molten salt bath. Laboratories usually immerse the edged lenses overnight so that they are ready for frame insertion the next day. The chemical formula of the salt bath for making photochromics impact-resistant varies from that of conventional lenses, although the immersion time is the same. Laboratories therefore have two sets of chemical tempering equipment so that all glass lenses can be treated during the same time period.

The possibility of spontaneous breakage, resulting in injuries if the lens "explodes" while the patient is wearing the glasses, is a major problem with heat-treated lenses. While this has not been known to occur with a chemically tempered lens, the tendency exists if it is subjected to deep scratches extending beyond the ion-exchange layer. For this reason Corning Glass Works recommends tempering for 15 to 16 hours, although less time is needed to produce a lens meeting the FDA regulation.

Unlike heat-treated lenses, those that are chemically strengthened can be resurfaced to make a small prescription change or to remove minor scratches. To make the lenses impact-resistant again, reprocessing in the salt bath is required.

If a coated lens is placed in the molten salt bath, the color coating and/or the antireflection coating are removed by the chemical. Coatings have to be applied after tempering has taken place. A tinted lens that owes its color to an oxide added to the ingredients of clear glass can be chemically tempered without affecting its appearance or seriously changing the absorptive properties of the color. (There is a very slight alteration in the IR end of the spectrum.)

Although a verifying certificate accompanies the lenses with the chemical-tempering process, there are few ways to test for the procedure. When viewed under the polariscope, some high plus, chemically tempered lenses exhibit a shape similar to a Maltese cross, but other chemically tempered lenses are free of a distinguishing pattern. This should not pose a problem since optical laboratories keep records for the FDA. Robert B. Pomeranz explained a possible testing procedure in the January 1977 issue of the *Optical Journal and Review of Optometry,* but practitioners are highly unlikely to test chemically tempered lenses in their offices. The procedure is as follows:

> Use an −11.00D uncut, 55mm round lens. Since it's uncut, it's also annealed and shows no contaminating stress pattern in the polarizer. It is also deep enough for this technique. Pour some glycerine into this −11.00D lens, hold it horizontally in the polarizer and then put one edge of the chem-temp lens to be tested in the fluid. If it has been chemically tempered, the edge will glow; an untreated lens won't glow. A bit of experience will enable you to distinguish chem-tempered lenses from untreated lenses. Moreover, the method is simple and precludes submerging the entire lens. We recommend keeping the glycerine in the bottle in order to keep it clean and undiluted with water when it's not being used. Glycerine may be hygroscopic and pull moisture out of the air.

Heat-treated (Air-treated) Lenses.   Before the introduction of chemically strengthened ophthalmic lenses, glass lenses were made impact-resistant by the heat-treating method. Such lenses exhibited serious drawbacks. Heat tempering consists of heating the glass lens almost to the point of melting and then cooling it quickly by a blast of air—thus the procedure is sometimes called "air tempering." This causes the surfaces to contract, building up pressures that should make the lens harder and stronger. However, if it is not properly heat-treated, or if it is scratched, the lens is less impact-resistant than an untreated lens and also becomes prone to what the optical industry refers to as "spontaneous breakage." In other words, the lens can shatter without an apparent foreign stress. The results can be disastrous if the breakage occurs while the patient is wearing the glasses. This confusion is eloquently described in an article by Barbara Katz that appeared in the *National Observer;*

> I had been browsing . . . when suddenly I heard a sharp cracking noise, felt something hit my right eye and I screamed. When I gingerly opened my eyes, I found myself staring at a crazy-quilt world. The right lens of my glasses had burst for no apparent reason. . . . small splinters dusted my face and some it seemed had entered my right eye.

The American Optometric Association has designed a card imprint, explaining that heat-treated lenses should be replaced if they become scratched. However, a far superior procedure would be the elimination of heat-treated lenses and the prescribing of plastic or chemically tempered lenses. There are no cases on record where the latter have spontaneously broken on the patient's face.

As a result of the heating and cooling procedure, all heat-treated lenses show some surface defacement that affects optical quality. This warpage can be seen by tilting the lens slightly while holding it out about 6 inches.

Weight can be a problem where heat-treated lenses are involved. To pass the drop-ball test as outlined in the FDA ruling, optical manufacturers have learned that the lens must have a 2.2mm minimum thickness, except in cases of high plus, where the thick center allows for a slight deviation. Chemically tempered lenses always meet the FDA standards in a thinner form.

Note: Most manufacturers in the United States use chemical tempering for plano lenses in sunglass designs; unfortunately, however, since the FDA finds heat-treating an acceptable procedure, many foreign manufacturers export lenses made "impact-resistant" by this method.

Occupational Protective Lenses

By definition, an impact-resistant occupational lens is one designed for industrial use. The original standard was as follows: a lens having 3.0mm minimum thickness with the exception of strong plus powers for which 2.5mm minimum thickness was considered adequate. In the test for strength, a 1⅛-inch steel ball is dropped freely from a height of 50 inches to the horizontal surface of the lens. Most manufacturers have discontinued 3.0mm minimum thickness hard resin because the added thickness is not needed to comply with the testing standards. Research also shows it to be unnecessary for chemically tempered lenses. "Occupational thickness" is a term primarily used when referring to extra-thick, heat-treated glass lenses.

The same heat-treating procedure is used as that involving thinner lenses. After the lens is edged to the desired size and shape, it is brought close to the melting point and then cooled rapidly so that tension is set up between the inner and outer molecular layers of glass. The additional lens thickness usually insures against spontaneous breakage, but the added weight makes it difficult to adjust the glasses comfortably and/or maintain a proper fit.

Many industries still supply these lenses, particularly in plano form. Workers often object to the unsightly appearance as well as the discomfort, so manufacturers try to solve some of the problems by limiting the patient's selection to a maximum eyesize of 48 or 50mm. However, their purpose may be defeated, because the small size subtracts from the protective value of the eyewear. In addition, as with all heat-treated lenses, there is surface defacement as a result of curvature distortion. Inexpensive industrial glasses may exhibit this excessively, because tight quality control is not always exercised in their manufacture.

Sometimes patients, particularly women, request industrial lenses be reshaped into a "better-looking" frame. Heat-treated lenses cannot be re-edged without danger of crumbling (2.2mm heat-treated lenses should never be reworked because of the increased possibility of spontaneous breakage). The best answer to this problem is the use of plastic lenses mounted into attractive frames. More industries are recognizing this logic and are issuing comfortable, well-fitting eyefashions to their employees.

Note: At one time, 2.0- to 2.2mm minimum thickness, heat-treated lenses were referred to as junior case-hardened or dress-hardened lenses; the industrial thickness lenses were called senior case-hardened or simply case-hardened lenses. Chemical tempering has rendered these terms obsolete.

Fresnel Lenses

The Fresnel lens is actually a plastic membrane, approximately 1mm thick, designed to be attached to an existing conventional plastic or glass lens. It is available in prismatic corrections, plus, and minus powers (see full discussion in Chapter 11, "Lenses for Special Uses"). Flexible when held in the hands (it is delivered in a special cardboard holder), the Fresnel membrane is not suitable for wear without the support of another lens. The press-on membrane is placed on the concave surface, using water, which provides enough suction to hold it in place. When attached to a glass lens, the glass does not have to be made impact-resistant. If breakage occurs, the Fresnel membrane "holds" the broken pieces. This characteristic simplifies their use for patients undergoing vision therapy. Fresnel lenses are used primarily as loaners intended for short-term wear. Often a number of prescription changes are needed within a short period and the Fresnel lens can be quickly attached to a non-impact-resistant lens.

Laminated Lenses

Laminated lenses may feature two relatively thin glass lenses bonded together by a cement-type material. There is also a laminated Corning lens called Corlon that bonds glass and plastic. The glass does not have to be made impact-resistant by heat treating or chemical tempering. If breakage occurs, all or most of the fragments are held intact by the bonding material.

Before the availability of chemical tempering, laminated lenses were used more frequently because they offered several advantages over heat-treated lenses. Since they are not subjected to the heating and cooling procedures, the ophthalmic curves remain true. In addition, spontaneous breakage is not a problem, so safety is a consideration in prescribing.

They were also used to obtain uniform color when a deeply tinted, high-power correction was needed. Before the widespread use of colored plastic lenses and glass coatings, most tinted lenses were the result of adding the proper oxide to the ingredients of clear glass. After the tinted blank was readied, the lens was ground to the desired prescription. In minus corrections this produced a lighter center; for a plus prescription the center was darker than the edges; high cylindrical powers resulted in color bands. These color differences became more obvious as the power and/or the size of the lenses increased. To counteract this problem, practitioners prescribed laminated lenses having a plano tinted lens bonded to one in clear with the proper prescription. (Superior methods of obtaining uniformity for tinted lenses are described in Chapter 9, "Prescribing Absorptive Lenses.")

Laminated lenses, except in Polaroid, have been phased out by most manufacturers. They had a tendency to split apart and with some high prescriptions, particularly those of minus power; the manufacturing process was too complicated to be feasible. Smaller eyesizes were necessary for comfort (because of the added thickness) and did not always offer adequate protection against the harmful rays of the sun.

Polaroid Laminated Lenses

By the nature of their construction, all Polaroid lenses meet the criteria set by the FDA ruling. Those of ophthalmic quality utilize either plastic or glass lenses, between which a polarizing material is sandwiched. The glass form does not need tempering because broken particles tend to be held intact by the Polaroid filter.

CONCLUSION

Although chemically tempered lenses have proven to be as impact resistant as those of hard-resin plastic, breakage could result in bits of broken glass becoming imbedded in the eye and surrounding facial tissue.

This could result in serious injury. Therefore, there are patients for whom it is critical that plastic lenses be recommended. In some cases polycarbonates are best as they are considered unbreakable.

1. **Monocular patients.** Patients having good vision in only one eye must be prescribed polycarbonate lenses. Since ocular trauma can readily result in blindness, all precautions must be taken, regardless of how slight the likelihood of accidental injury.

2. **Children who wear glasses all or most waking hours.** By nature children are extremely active and often unaware of potential danger that might result in ocular injury. Polycarbonate lenses offer the utmost in safety and comfort.

3. **Patients involved in hazardous occupations.** Large industries recognizing the hazardous aspects of various plant operations require impact-resistant lenses. Almost without exception, insurance coverage for employees hinges on the wearing of specific types of eyewear whenever and wherever it is deemed necessary. However, there are patients, usually self-employed, who do not recognize or acknowledge the possibility of on-the-job ocular injury. It is important, therefore, that the practitioner explore all phases of a patient's occupational and avocational needs so that plastic lenses can be prescribed if a hazard exists.

4. **Any patient concerned about possible eye complications.** It is not unusual for a practitioner to counsel patients overly concerned about the likelihood of ocular injury. In these cases, prescribing polycarbonate lenses is an assurance that the best protection has been provided.

A particularly interesting research project, the results of which were published in the June 1968 issue of the *American Journal of Optometry* and in the *Archives of the American Academy of Optometry*, presented another reason for recommending plastic lenses. Titled "Delayed Flaking from Scratches in Glass" and authored by physicist Barry A. J. Clark, the phenomenon presented was that a glass lens does not have to break to be hazardous—scratching alone can present a problem. By the use of microscopic photographs, the delayed-action ejection of small sharp-edged fragments from scratches in glass was studied. It was noted that these fragments are ejected with sufficient velocity to travel to the eyes of spectacle wearers. Although the glass fragments from a scratch on the ocular surface were expelled with velocities much smaller than necessary for penetration into the eyeball, the fragments could lodge between the eyelid and the conjunctiva. Eye movements and blinking would therefore result in abrasion and consequent risk of infection. In addition, the fragments are difficult to remove because of their transparency and small size.

Under the same testing conditions, scratches on a CR 39 plastic lens did not result in a delayed-action ejection of fragments.

In conclusion the author stated; "It should be clearly understood that the hazard present is of a relatively minor nature when compared with the type and frequency of eye hazards found and is therefore not to be regarded as justification for the nonuse of glass safety spectacles." Nevertheless, the implications are obvious. When the practitioner prescribes an impact-resistant lens, it is the plastic designs that prove the most effective.

Chapter 11

LENSES FOR SPECIAL USES

INTRODUCTION

There are lens designs that, although limited in use, often serve an important role in the fabrication of eyewear. In some instances they are superior to conventional lenses, resulting in better cosmetic and/or optical performance.

FRESNEL MEMBRANE PRESS-ON LENSES

The Fresnel press-on membrane is a thin plastic sheet of about 1mm designed to be placed on the ocular surface of an existing glass or plastic lens. It is available in prism corrections, plus and minus full lenses, and a precut plus power ST25mm bifocal-style. Application is quick and simple; water is the only substance needed to hold the membrane in place.

Originally distributed by Optical Science Group, Inc., Fresnel lenses are available from Mentor and obtained through the local laboratory. The membrane is supplied in a squared cardboard carrier. It can be shaped with a scissors or by means of specially designed cutting equipment to conform to an existing lens.

Fresnel lenses are rarely worn as a permanent correction because they exhibit several problems. Visual acuity is usually reduced one line by Fresnel optics and all result in a cosmetic loss. Yet, they can serve important roles, as is explained under each type of correction. Since increment steps have varied in the past, it is best to query the laboratory as to availability.

Fresnel Press-on Prisms

The optical principle of the prism corrections involves the use of a series of small prisms of equal power whose bases are arranged parallel to each other. The result is a series of parallel lines noticed by both wearer and observer. Fresnel prism powers range from $\frac{1}{2}^\Delta$ to 30^Δ diopters. Unusual prism prescriptions formerly difficult or impossible to fabricate are now easily available by using the Fresnel press-on membrane. Examples include prism power in bifocal segments and sectional application of prism (i.e., prism in a portion of the lens compensating for a palsied extraocular muscle). Large amounts of prism, such as 15 diopters or greater, can be tolerated since the total eyewear weight is as though no significant prismatic correction was worn. However, as with all Fresnel optics, there is a loss of visual acuity, and cosmesis is adversely affected. These lenses are used primarily as temporary corrections during vision-training therapy. Practitioners who specialize in this field find them invaluable in evaluating quickly the amount of prism best serving the patient's needs. Changing the correction is a relatively low-cost procedure, and it takes only minutes to shape the membrane to an existing lens.

Fresnel Membrane Press-on Plus Full Lenses

These lenses are easily available in powers +0.50D through +20.00D, with the design involving a series of concentric circles. The lower plus powers are used primarily as aids in vision training but the reduction of visual acuity limits their practicability. The high powers offer an interim lens, quickly obtained for the aphakic patient whose final correction has not been determined.

Fresnel Precut ST25mm Plus Segments

These add powers ranging from +0.50D to +8.00D can help evaluate the patient's need for a specific near correction. The higher powers can provide an inexpensive low vision aid, but the resultant drop in visual acuity hinders their value.

Fresnel Minus Lenses

Minus Fresnel lenses range in power from −1.00D to −14.00D and exhibit a concentric ring pattern. They are sometimes used in vision-training procedures but tend to be more practical as "loaners" to the myope who cannot function without a correction during the time it takes the laboratory to fabricate conventional eyewear.

HIGH ADD BIFOCALS FOR LOW VISION PATIENTS

Patients whose best corrected visual acuity is less than 20/50 may require bifocal adds higher than the +3.50D usually available from the local laboratory. Any conventional fused or one-piece bifocal can be factory ordered with a high add; the upper limit is usually +8.00D, although the manufacturer should be queried since there is a slight variation for each style.

There are special lenses exclusively designed for the low vision patient. Designs for Vision, Inc., located in New York City, offers a high add CR 39 lens. These Franklin-style bifocals look like the Executive lens and have add powers ranging from +4.00D to +20.00D. These are also available in Executive trifocal form. Since these are cemented segments, they may be ordered with any intermediate and near powers. Prism can be incorporated if necessary.

In addition, it is possible to order cemented segments placed on single-vision lenses. They are usually fixed on the inside surface but can be ordered on the outside curvature. The segments can be either glass or plastic, but fusion of glass to plastic is not recommended. Currently used plastic cements do not discolor and dry up with age as they did in the past. There are a number of advantages in prescribing cemented segments. The most important is versatility, because the segment can be ordered in any size and design (round-top, flat-top, or straight-across), with any amount of prism in cases where fusion is a problem.

However, most practitioners prefer using the cemented Franklin-style lenses from Designs for Vision, Inc., because local laboratories are often not familiar with the procedures necessary to produce a quality cement-segment bifocal.

American Optical makes available special molded one-piece, front surface high add powers for the aphakic low vision patient. The present range is +6.00 to +8.00D adds, with exact increments obtained by querying the manufacturer.

HIGH-INDEX GLASS LENSES

The original high-index lenses, usually identified as Thinlite or Flintlite, were fashioned of flint glass. Flint has an index of 1.7, so the lenses were thinner than those of standard crown and were recommended for high minus corrections. However, they exhibited several problems. Since flint was relatively heavy, the eyewear tended to be very uncomfortable. In addition, the extreme chromatic aberration and resultant color distortion often annoyed the wearer. Flint lenses were brittle, tending to break more readily than crown. In fact, the FDA ruling regarding impact-resistant lenses made it almost impossible to prescribe them. They could not be made impact-resistant, and practitioners fearful of lawsuits hesitated about asking the patient to sign a waiver.

A high-index 1.7 lens eliminating many of the problems of Flintlite has been introduced. Designed primarily for high minus prescriptions, the weight is about that of crown and actually less when the power reaches greater than −8.00D. The lens can be made impact-resistant by the chemical-tempering method. A special design, LHI (lightweight, high index), developed by Hoya Lens has such a low color-dispersion factor that it is comparable to crown glass.

A number of lens manufacturers now make high-index 1.6, 1.7, and 1.8 glass lenses. However, when thin-appearing lenses are critical to the patient needing −6.00D and greater, the high-index plastic polycarbonate designs are probably a better solution. Although not as thin looking, they are much more comfortable and cosmetically very acceptable.

X-RAY GLASS LENS

Vision-Ease makes available a high-index 1.8 clear lens manufactured of flint glass for use around radiology equipment. This lens cannot be made impact resistant by chemical treating or heat tempering, so the patient must sign a waiver before it is prescribed. Specifics can be obtained by querying the manufacturer.

LENSES FOR THE APHAKIC PATIENT

Determining the most suitable lens design for the aphakic patient is a critical consideration (this discussion obviously does not include the pseudophake with an implant lens needing a relatively low prescription). Since the correction is high plus in power, weight is an important factor. When the patient looks away from the optical centers of the lenses, the prismatic effect can result in asthenopia. Cosmesis is always a problem. Facial features viewed through the correction appear considerably magnified and, therefore, distorted.

Whenever possible, contact lenses should be fit to the aphake. The drawbacks resulting from wearing high plus spectacle lenses are either eliminated or considerably minimized. There is. however, always the need for conventional eyewear because few aphakic patients can wear contact lenses comfortably for more than 10 to 12 hours a day. There are also times when contacts cannot be worn because the patient has a cold or influenza or is otherwise indisposed.

There are important advances in the design of hard-resin aphakic lenses. The wide-angle designs, which essentially duplicate the optics of a lenticular style while dramatically improving cosmesis (the lenses look conventional), are the finest available for the high plus patient. They are called Welsh 4-Drop Aspherics (designed by R. C. Welsh) because there is approximately four diopters less power in the periphery, allowing certain areas of the face to appear more normal. The lenses also give the patient a wider distant field of view. While there may be a drop in visual acuity unless the head is turned, it is less than that resulting from the distortion of full high plus lenses. In actuality there is a certain amount of compensation because of the change in vertex distance. Plus powers increase in effectivity when positioned further away from the pupil, so the periphery has more power than indicated by the lensometer.

Welsh 4-Drop Aspherics are available in a single-vision and two bifocal styles. The straight-top D design has a segment size 22 × 11mm, the shorter vertical measurement designed to allow the patient to see beneath the segment for better orientation when walking, climbing stairs, etc. The other bifocal design is the round-top 22mm, having its widest area 11mm below the segment line. Since most aphakic patients are geriatric persons with a "touch" of arthritis in the neck area, the latter is not practical. It is difficult to hold the head in a relatively normal position for lengthy reading with any pleasure.

There is also available a 3-Drop aspheric lens similar in basic construction to the Welsh 4-Drop, except that the power difference from center to edge is about 3 diopters. The straight-top D segment is the conventional 22mm × 14mm; the practitioner may prefer prescribing it for the larger reading area. The basic advantages are the same for both designs.

Lenses designed for the aphakic patient that feature a round lenticular field are obsolete. Armorlite manufactures a CR 39 lenticular lens superior in appearance to the older versions. Rather than the traditional 38 or 40mm round lenticular area (Figures 11.1 and 11.2), the OV-AL has a usable oval-shaped 45mm × 40mm field (Figure 11.3). It comes in single-vision and two bifocal styles; the round-top 22mm, and the conventional straight-top D 22mm segment.

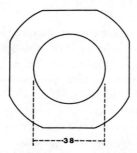

FIGURE 11.1   *Lenticular lens—38mm prescription area*

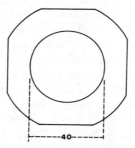

FIGURE 11.2   *Lenticular lens—40mm prescription area*

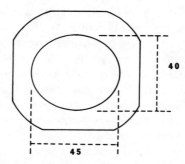

FIGURE 11.3   *45 × 40mm oval lenticular field*

However, the Welsh 4-Drop and the 3-Drop plastic CR 39 aspheric lenses combine the best optics with excellent cosmesis (there are no lines separating distant power areas) and are the finest available cataract lenses. They can be tinted for an out-of-doors prescription in any desired shade. A separate dark pair should be prescribed in addition to the plano sun-lenses worn with contacts, since almost all aphakic patients are extremely photophobic.

If the aphakic patient enjoys close-work activities for long periods of time, it is also best to recommend a near single-vision correction in addition to bifocals. This should not be a drop-design in order to make full plus available through the lower portion of the lens.

Some manufacturers of glass lenses either make specially designed cataract lenses or state that their conventional lenses are suitable for the aphakic patient. Glass lenses should not be prescribed in high plus corrections. Even when lens size is kept to a minimum, it is almost impossible to make the eyewear comfortable.

BLENDED MYODISC (YOUNGER OPTICS)

Recently available is a hard-resin CR 39 minus power lens from Younger Optics that is designed for cosmetic purposes. Edge thickness is reduced by about 40%. The design is similar to the 4-Drop aspheric lens for plus prescriptions, basically a lenticular without the lenticular ledges. This means that the peripheral areas are not ground to full power. Blended myodisc lenses are available in powers ranging from −4.00D sphere to −28.00D sphere. The spherical component is combined with cylinder power up to −2.00D only, but this range may be expanded. The lens is also made with special UV absorbers that give specific colors identified as PLS 400, PLS 530, PLS 540, and PLS 550. See Chapter 9, "Prescribing Absorptive Lenses" for specifics.

It may be well to know that some local laboratories use exclusive names for the Blended Myodisc lenses, e.g., Thin-Rex.

Note: The old Myodisc with a "scooped-out" field and peripheral plano surfaces front and back of the lens should never be recommended. Blended Myodisc lenses look "normal" and offer superior cosmetic/comfort properties.

BASE CURVE
CONSIDERATIONS

INTRODUCTION

Perhaps the most confusing and controversial subject in lens design prescribing is the specification of base curves. There are practitioners who rarely designate a base curve on a lens prescription. They feel that the designer's academic background and extensive research in the field of ophthalmic optics has resulted in lenses having optimum optical performance. In fact, many laboratories will not deviate from the recommended base curves suggested by the manufacturers, especially when oversize, plastic, or photochromic lenses are involved. Sometimes it is a certainty that the ordered curves would adversely affect cosmetic value. In other instances grinding certain curvatures on some lens designs is a procedure too complicated to be feasible. This chapter will discuss the options open to the practitioner as well as changes that have occurred regarding base curves.

BASE CURVES OF SINGLE-VISION LENSES

If a single-vision lens is spherical in correction, the base curve is that curvature common to a series (see Chapter 1, "Characteristics of Lenses"). This definition has remained constant for decades, but within the past few years defining the base curve for a cylindrical lens has been changing. Most manufacturers are phasing out plus cylinder, single-vision lenses and discarding the definition that the base curve is the weakest curve on the cylinder surface. Almost without exception, the preferred definition for a minus cylinder design is that the base curve is the spherical (outside) curvature of the lens.

Every major glass lens manufacturer distributes single-vision and conventional multifocal lenses having specific base curves that correct for certain lens aberrations. At one time local laboratories stocked at least one brand in both plus and minus cylinder corrections, but in the United States the plus cylinder series are phased out.

Optical experts prefer minus cylinder lenses because a spherical front surface means that meridional magnification is kept at a minimum. Cosmetic appearance is more pleasing also because curvature changes are on the back surface and therefore less noticeable.

The beginning presbyope who has worn a single-vision inside surface cylinder design usually makes the transition from single-vision to bifocal lenses with relative ease. All contemporary multifocals manufactured in the United States (glass and plastic) are made in minus cylinder form.

TRADE NAMES FOR GLASS LENSES HAVING SPECIFIC BASE CURVE CONSTRUCTION

The following identification is given primarily for historical purposes and because reference in texts is still made to these trade names. Manufacturers often used the term "corrected curve" when referring to quality glass lenses. It has largely been dropped in reference to plastic lenses because it is assumed that all are designed for optimum performance/ cosmetic value.

Orthogon Lenses.   The Orthogon series of corrected curve lenses was introduced by Bausch & Lomb, Inc., in 1928. The lenses were ground on any one of 15 base curves, depending on the prescription. All the original designs featured a toric front surface and corrected for radial astigmatism but not for curvature of field.

Tillyer Lenses. The original Tillyer lenses were introduced in 1926 by American Optical Corp. These lenses were ground in plus cylinder form with the exception of a few minus powers that had a back cylinder design. They featured a partial correction of both marginal astigmatism and curvature of field. The Tillyer name is retained to designate quality lens designs.

Tillyer Masterpiece. In 1964 the Tillyer Masterpiece lens series was introduced. These lenses are ground in minus cylinder form and keep meridional magnification at a minimum.

Kurova Lenses. This corrected curve series was created by Continental Optical Co. Ground in plus toric form, they were designed to keep marginal astigmatism at a minimum. The term "Kurova" now is used by Shuron-Textron to mean quality lenses.

Shursite Lenses. These lenses were made available in 1966 by Shuron/ Continental (now Shuron-Textron) Optical Co. They were ground in minus cylinder form and designed to keep meridional magnification at a minimum. Kurova is now the reference name for such lenses.

Normalsite Lenses. Normalsite lenses, distributed by Titmus Optical Co., were originally manufactured in plus cylinder form and later replaced by a minus cylinder construction.

Note: Uni-form lenses created by Univis, Inc., and later distributed under the trade name Best-Form were one of the first minus cylinder designs with meridional magnification kept at a minimum. They were discontinued in 1971.

BASE CURVE OF MULTIFOCALS

The base curve of a multifocal is identified as the spherical distance curvature on the same side as the segment. For all U.S. contemporary designs this is the convex (outside) surface of the lens. Specific curvatures can be ascertained by charts available from the various manufacturers. If conventional glass multifocals are prescribed and a different curvature is requested, the base curve can often be altered. The process is more difficult with plastic lenses and few local laboratories will deviate from the manufacturer's designations.

POSSIBLE DEVIATIONS FROM SUGGESTED BASE CURVES

All quality laboratories have trained technicians who can determine what curves will give the best optical and cosmetic effect for a given prescription. As has been previously noted, it is becoming increasingly difficult for the practitioner to deviate from these recommendations, yet there are times when attempts to do so may be necessary.

If the lens powers for a given prescription are drastically different for each eye, specifying that the outside curves be approximately the same is a critical cosmetic factor.

A practitioner may feel that when a patient has adjusted to specific base curves, curvatures should be duplicated. However, with today's lens and frame designs, this theory is difficult to follow. If glasses have been worn, particularly those having a high correction, when the curves are changed, the patient should be advised of the possibility of an adjustment period (usually a few weeks). Some patients are sensitive to changes in base curve if they alternate between more than one pair. For example, a patient may wear an outdoor correction having plastic lenses and an indoor prescription utilizing glass lenses. The curvatures may not be the same. Whenever possible, it is best to recommend lenses with similar base curves.

A problem can arise from the use of minus cylinder, single-vision glass lenses. Since they are ground with flatter curves than plus cylinder designs, the patient with long lashes and/or a flat bridge may find that the lashes touch the lenses. A deeper lens can be ordered (i.e., +8.00 or +9.00D outside curvature), but this often means sacrificing cosmetic appearance. Fortunately, many attractive contemporary frames are available with an adjustable pad bridge construction so that they can be positioned properly; alternatively, the patient may prefer to slide the eyewear slightly down the nose.

It is wise to clock lenses with the Geneva Lens Gauge when the eyewear is received from the laboratory and record the base curves. Sometimes a change in curvature is a continuing annoyance to the patient; such knowledge is helpful when pinpointing possible sources of problems. In very rare cases it may be necessary to change back to lenses duplicating the original base curves.

BALANCE LENS

It may be well to mention here the ordering of a balance lens for the patient whose vision cannot be improved in one eye. If "balance lens" is written on the prescription form, the laboratory may use any available discarded lens. For cosmetic effect the balance lens should be ordered close to the prescription for the other eye and in the same lens design. Eyewear is not attractive if, for instance, the patient wears an ST25mm D-style bifocal before the right eye and a single-vision lens in front of the left.

FRONT SURFACE CURVATURE AND LENS MAGNIFICATION

There may be instances when the practitioner wishes to know the magnification created by a lens. Magnification or image size depends upon four factors. The first of these factors is unalterable; the other three can be controlled.

1. Power of the lens
2. Front surface curvature (this variable contributes the most to magnification effects)
3. Lens thickness
4. Vertex distance

Magnification is computed using the following formulas:

$$M_p = \frac{1}{1 - hD_v}$$

M_p = magnification as a result of the power

$$M_s = \frac{1}{1 - D_1(t/n)}$$

h = vertex distance
D_v = vertex power
M_s = magnification as a result of the shape of the lens
D_1 = power of the front curve
t = thickness in meters of the lens
n = index of the lens

$$M_{total} = M_p \times M_s$$

$$M_{total} = \text{total magnification}$$

$$\% = (M_{total} - 1) \times 100\%$$

The answer is stated in percentage of magnification.

PROBLEM:

A 45mm round lens of +2.00D power is worn 16mm anterior to the cornea. This lens has a +8.00D front surface, a −6.00D ocular surface, and is 2.5mm thick (center position). What is the magnification produced by the lens?

PROCEDURE:

1.   Determine the magnification as a result of the power.

$$M_p = \frac{1}{1 - hD_v}$$

$$= \frac{1}{1 - (0.016)(+2)}$$

$$= 1.03$$

2.   Determine the magnification because of the shape.

$$M_s = \frac{1}{1 - (t/n)\, D_1}$$

$$= \frac{1}{1 - (0.0025/1.523)(8)}$$

$$= 1.01$$

3.   Determine total magnification.

$$M_{total} = M_p \times M_s$$
$$= 1.03 \times 1.01$$
$$= 1.04$$

4. $\% = (M_{total} - 1) \times 100\%$
$$= (1.04 - 1) \times 100\%$$
$$= 4\%$$

SOLUTION:

Magnification = 4%.

PROBLEM:

What is the magnification of a +3.00D spherical lens constructed with a +6.00D front surface and center thickness of 2mm, and worn with the back vertex 17mm from the entrance pupil of the eye?

PROCEDURE:

1. Determine the magnification as a result of the power.

$$M_p = \frac{1}{1 - (0.017)(+3)}$$
$$= 1.05$$

2. Determine the magnification because of the shape.

$$M_s = \frac{1}{1 - (0.002/1.523)(6)}$$
$$= \frac{1}{0.992}$$
$$= 1.008$$

3. Determine the total magnification.

$$M_{total} = 1.05 \times 1.008$$
$$= 1.058$$

4. $\% = (M_{total} - 1) \times 100\%$
    $= (1.058 - 1) \times 100\%$
    $= 5.8\%$

SOLUTION:

Magnification = 5.8%.

If a practitioner wishes to equalize the magnification of two lenses, it can be done by changing the front curvature of one lens. Two problems follow as examples of how this is accomplished.

PROBLEM:

A patient wears a pair of spectacles 15mm anterior to the corneal vertex. The left lens is a +2.00D sphere with 2.5mm center thickness. The right lens is +3.00D with 3.0mm center thickness and has a front curvature of +6.00D. The index of the lenses is 1.52. Determine the front curvature of the left lens if both lenses are to have equal magnification.

1.   Determine magnification of the right lens.

$$M_p = \frac{1}{1 - hD_v}$$

$$= \frac{1}{1 - (0.015)(3)} = \frac{1}{0.955}$$

$$= 1.046$$

$$M_s = \frac{1}{1 - t/n \ (D_1)}$$

$$= \frac{1}{1 - (0.003/1.52)(6)} = \frac{1}{0.988}$$

$$= 1.01$$

$$M_{total} = 1.046 \times 1.01 = 1.056$$
$$\% = (1.056 - 1.00) \times 100\% = 5.6\%$$

2.   Determine magnification as a result of the power of the left lens.

$$M_p = \frac{1}{1 - hD_v}$$

$$= \frac{1}{1 - (0.015)(2)} = \frac{1}{0.97}$$

$$= 1.03$$

3.   Determine magnification needed from shape factor for the right lens.

$$M_{total} = M_p \times M_s$$

$$M_s = \frac{1.056}{1.03}$$

$$= 1.02$$

4.   Solve for front curvature of right lens.

$$M_s = \frac{1}{1 - t/n \ (D_1)}$$

$$1.02 = \frac{1}{1 - (0.0025/1.52) \ D_1}$$

$$1.02 - 0.00163 \ D_1 = 1$$
$$0.00163 \ D_1 = 0.02$$
$$D_1 = +12.00D$$

SOLUTION:

Front surface of left lens needs to be $+12.00D$ to equalize magnification.

PROBLEM:

A patient requires the following prescription:

$$O.D. + 4.00 \text{ D. S.}$$
$$O.S. + 3.00 \text{ D. S.}$$

The center thickness of the right lens is 3.5mm. The front curve is $+10.00D$. The center thickness of the left lens is 3.5mm. The lens index is 1.52; the vertex distance is 12mm. Calculate the front curvature of the left lens necessary to equalize the magnification.

1. Determine M_{total} for right lens.

$$M_p = \frac{1}{1 - hD_v}$$

$$= \frac{1}{1 - (0.012)(4)} = \frac{1}{0.952}$$

$$= 1.05$$

$$M_s = \frac{1}{1 - t/n \, (D_1)}$$

$$= \frac{1}{1 - (0.0035/1.52)(10)} = \frac{1}{0.977}$$

$$= 1.02$$

$$M_{total} = 1.05 \times 1.02 = 1.07$$
$$\% = (1.07 - 1.00) \times 100\%$$
$$= 7\%$$

2. Determine M_p for left lens.

$$M_p = \frac{1}{1 - hD_v}$$

$$= \frac{1}{1 - (0.012)(3)} = \frac{1}{0.964}$$

$$= 1.03$$

3. Determine M_s for left lens.

$$M_s = \frac{1.07}{1.03}$$

$$= 1.04$$

4. Determine D_1 for left lens.

$$1.04 = \frac{1}{1 - (0.0035/1.52)\, D_1}$$

$$1.04 - 0.0024\, D_1 = 1$$
$$0.0024\, D_1 = 0.04$$
$$D_1 = +16.66D$$

SOLUTION:

The front curvature of the left lens needs to be $+16.62D$ (the closest $0.12D$) to equalize magnification.

Chapter 13

VERTICAL IMBALANCE AT THE READING LEVEL

INTRODUCTION

When a patient looks beneath the distance optical centers of lenses having different powers in the vertical meridians, prismatic imbalance results. If the imbalance is 1½ prism diopters or more, the practitioner needs to be aware of possible symptoms, such as a pulling sensation "when I read," doubling when reading, and/or headaches usually in the frontal area.

Vertical prismatic imbalance can be eliminated or considerably reduced by a number of methods, the most satisfactory of which is bicentric grinding (slab-off). Bicentric grinding is the only possible procedure when a single-vision correction is involved. Until 1986, the two optical centers were created in the lens having the highest minus or lowest plus power (to counteract the prism base-down effect). Then Younger Optics introduced a plastic CR 39, slab-off, molded with prism base down on the front surface of the blank. It is placed on the most plus (least minus) lens. Both methods result in a slab-off line that extends from the temporal to the nasal extremities of the lens. Its appearance is similar to that of a straight-across bifocal, and its height is determined in the same manner as that of a conventional straight-top bifocal (usually 1mm below the lower lid).

Vertical prismatic imbalance in a bifocal correction can be compensated for by the slab-off procedure either by the conventional method or by Younger Optics' reverse slab-off (made in Flat-top 25mm and 28mm). Prescribing bifocal segments having optical centers varying in position or using segments having the compensating prism ground into them is also possible, but these two methods have been made obsolete by the efficiency of bicentric grinding (also known as the slab-off procedure).

When it is necessary to compensate for vertical prismatic imbalance in a trifocal correction, the conventional slab-off method is the only possible procedure (placed on the highest minus).

BICENTRIC GRINDING IN A SINGLE-VISION PRESCRIPTION

It is rare to correct for vertical imbalance in a single-vision prescription. Usually the patient is instructed to hold reading material in a relatively straightforward position. This enables the patient to look just below the optical centers of the lenses when focusing at the near point.

In cases where the patient's visual tasks do not make this possible, a slab-off correction is prescribed. To determine the amount it is first necessary to compute the vertical prismatic imbalance at the reading level. It is assumed that the patient reads 8mm below the distance optical centers of the lenses unless otherwise measured.

PROBLEM:

A patient requires the following prescription:
O.D. +4.00D.S.
O.S. +1.00D.S.
A decision is made to prescribe a slab-off lens. How would this correction be ordered from the laboratory?

PROCEDURE:

1. The formula for determining vertical imbalance is the Prentice Prism Formula.

$$\text{Vertical imbalance} = F_v \text{ (cm)}$$

F_v = difference in power between the vertical meridians of the two lenses.

cm = distance from the optical centers of the lenses to the reading point.

2. vertical imbalance $= +4.00 - (+1.00) \times 0.8$cm
$$= 2.4^\Delta$$

3. Slab-off is ordered in $\frac{1}{2}^\Delta$ steps rounded off to the lowest half.

SOLUTION:

Slab-off 2^Δ O.S. at 14mm high (height arbitrarily determined for demonstration purpose).

SPECIAL NOTE:

If the Younger Optics reverse slab-off lenses (available in CR 39 only) were used, the slab-off correction would be 2^Δ on the *right* lens.

PROBLEM:

A patient wears the following correction:
O.D. $+6.00 -2.00 \times 45°$
O.S. $+2.00 -4.00 \times 30°$
If bicentric grinding were required, what would be ordered from the laboratory? The patient reads 7mm below the distance optical centers.

PROCEDURE:

1. Determine the power in the vertical meridian of each lens.

   O.D. $+6.00 + (\frac{1}{2})(-2.00) = +5.00$D
   O.S. $+2.00 + (\frac{3}{4})(-4.00) = -1.00$D

2. Determine the difference in lens power.

   $+5.00 - (-1.00) = 6.00$D

3. Compute the amount of vertical imbalance.

$$V.I. = F_v(cm)$$
$$= 6 \times 0.7$$
$$= 4.2^\Delta$$

Overcompensation is not desired, so the slab-off correction is rounded to the lowest $\frac{1}{2}$ prism diopter (ordered in $\frac{1}{2}$ prism diopter steps).

SOLUTION:

Slab-off 4^Δ O.S. at 14mm high (height arbitrarily determined for demonstration purposes).
   Note: The Younger Optics reverse slab-off correction is 4^Δ O.D.

PROBLEM:

Given the following prescription:

$$\text{O.D. } +3.00 -2.00 \times 45°$$
$$\text{O.S. } \text{plano } -4.00 \times 90°$$

If the patient reads 8mm below the distance optical centers, what is the slab-off correction ordered from the laboratory?

PROCEDURE:

1. Determine the power in the vertical meridian of each lens.

$$\text{O.D. } +3.00 + (\tfrac{1}{2})\,(-2.00) = +2.00D$$
$$\text{O.S. } \quad 0.00 + \quad (0)(-4.00) = 0.00D$$

2. Determine the difference in lens powers.

$$+2.00 -0.00 = 2.00D$$

3. Compute the amount of vertical imbalance.

$$\begin{aligned} \text{V.I.} &= F_v(\text{cm}) \\ &= 2\,(0.8) \\ &= 1.6^\Delta \end{aligned}$$

SOLUTION:

Slab-off 1.5^Δ O.S. (at measured height; i.e., 15mm high) or Younger Optics reverse slab-off, 1.5^Δ O.D.

Note: Practically speaking, this imbalance is too small to give rise to symptoms, so a correction is unnecessary.

PROBLEM:

The following lenses are prescribed

$$\text{O.D. } -1.00 -5.00 \times 180°$$
$$\text{O.S. } -2.00 \text{ D.S.}$$

The patient reads 7mm below the optical centers. How is the bicentric grinding ordered?

PROCEDURE:

1. Determine the power in the vertical meridian of each lens.

$$\text{O.D. } -1.00 + (1)\,(-5.00) = -6.00D$$
$$\text{O.S. } -2.00 \text{ D.S.}$$

2. Determine the difference in lens powers.

$$-6.00 - (-2.00) = -4.00D$$

3. Compute the vertical imbalance.

$$\begin{aligned} \text{V.I.} &= F_v(\text{cm}) \\ &= 4\,(.7) \\ &= 2.8^\Delta \end{aligned}$$

SOLUTION:

Slab-off 2.5^Δ O.D. (at the measured height; i.e., 14mm high) or 2.5^Δ O.S. for Younger Optics reverse slab-off.

SLAB-OFF IN A BIFOCAL PRESCRIPTION

There are a number of methods used to compensate for vertical imbalance at the reading level in a bifocal correction. The most practical method is the slab-off procedure. From a cosmetic viewpoint it is the most pleasing, because the slab-off line coincides with the segment dividing line. (A straight-top design, preferably ST25mm or 28mm, should be prescribed.)

When ordering bicentric grinding in a bifocal correction, the procedure is the same as that used with a single-vision correction. The add power at near does not affect the amount of vertical imbalance because it is the same for both eyes.

PROBLEM:

A patient wears the following prescription:

O.D. $+6.00 -2.00 \times 45°$
O.S. $+3.00 -2.00 \times 30°$
O.U. Add $+2.00D$

ST25 bifocal style set at 14mm high

If the patient reads 8mm below the distance optical centers, what would be the bicentric grinding ordered from the laboratory?

PROCEDURE:

1. Determine the power in the vertical meridian of each lens.

O.D. $+6.00 + (\frac{1}{2})\,(-2.00) = +5.00D$
O.S. $+3.00 + (\frac{3}{4})\,(-2.00) = +1.50D$

2.   Determine the vertical imbalance.

$$V.I. = (+5.00 - 1.50)\,(0.8)$$
$$= 2.8^{\Delta}$$

SOLUTION:

Slab-off 2.5^{Δ} O.S. at 14mm high to coincide with the segment height, or Younger Optics reverse slab-off 2.5^{Δ} O.D.

SLAB-OFF OR BICENTRIC GRINDING IN A TRIFOCAL CORRECTION

The amount of slab-off in a trifocal correction is computed and ordered in the same manner as that of a bifocal prescription. Since the intermediate and near adds are equal for each eye, the compensation is for the imbalance caused by the difference in distance power between the two lenses. A straight-top trifocal design should always be used. It is best to order the slab-off line coinciding with the division between the near and intermediate segments, although it can be placed at the separation between the intermediate and distance if desired.

PROBLEM:

A patient needs the following trifocal prescription:

$$O.D. -5.00 - .50 \times 180°$$
$$O.S. -2.00 - 1.50 \times 45°$$
$$O.U. \text{ Add } +2.50D$$

An ST7–28mm trifocal lens is prescribed with an overall segment height of 22mm. If the patient reads 12mm below the distance optical centers, what would be the bicentric grinding ordered from the laboratory?

SOLUTION:

1.   Determine the power in the vertical meridian of each lens.

$$O.D. -5.00 + (-0.50) = -5.50D$$
$$O.S. -2.00 + (½)(-1.00) = -2.50D$$

2.   Determine the difference in lens power.

$$-5.50 - (-2.50) = -3.00D$$

3. Compute the amount of vertical imbalance.

$$\text{V.I.} = F_v(\text{cm})$$
$$= 3 \times 1.2$$
$$= 3.6^\Delta$$

ANSWER:

Correction is rounded to the lowest ½ prism diopter; slab-off 3.5^Δ O.D. (highest minus) at 15mm high. Total segment height is 22mm; intermediate segment is 7mm high. Height of near segment is (22mm–7mm) or 15mm high; slab-off line will coincide with division between near and intermediate segments.

Note: As of this writing, Younger Optics does not manufacture a reverse slab-off trifocal.

Special Notes Regarding Bicentric Grinding (Slab-off Corrections)

1. Until recently, local laboratories designed and made most slab-off corrections. The result was high breakage and a slab-off line that often was "wavy." Vision-Ease now stocks conventional glass bicentric semifinished blanks in all straight-top segment styles. The slab-off line is always straight; there is faster service and a more reliable delivery date. Available powers are 1½ prism diopters to 6 prism diopters. Vision-Ease will also make any bicentric lens (power, tint, etc.) on special order and calculate the amount of prism if the practitioner desires that service. This includes Executive-type corrections, which many local laboratories hesitated to supply because of difficulty in processing.

2. The Younger slab-off series made in CR 39 only is available in 1½-prism diopter to 6-prism diopter corrections in single-vision and two bifocal styles, ST25mm and ST28mm. There are also special UV-absorbing lenses available. This excellent form of bicentric corrections must involve an explanation to the patient wearing a conventional slab-off lens; otherwise it is easy to assume that the correction was placed on the wrong lens.

3. The term "double slab-off" sometimes seen in texts does not apply to a correction for vertical imbalance. At one time this procedure was used to reduce lower edge thickness of high minus lenses, but the resultant slab-off lines on both lenses made the cosmetic value doubtful. High-

index plastic lenses now available are the recognized cosmetic solution.

CHECKING THE AMOUNT OF SLAB-OFF ON A LENS

When checking a slab-off prescription, the amount of bicentric grinding is easily determined by using the Geneva Lens Measure.

1. Place the three pins of the gauge horizontally on the surface with the bicentric grinding. They are positioned just above the slab-off line (Figure 13.1).
2. Note the reading on the gauge.
3. Hold the gauge vertically with the center pin on the slab-off line (Figure 13.2).
4. Note the reading on the gauge.
5. The difference between the two readings is the amount of bicentric grinding.

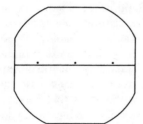
FIGURE 13.1   *Slab-off line*

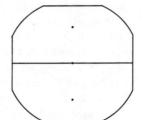
FIGURE 13.2   *Slab-off line*

Example

With the pins positioned horizontally the reading is +6.50D. The reading with the gauge held vertically is +10.00D. Therefore, the amount of slab-off is $3\frac{1}{2}^\Delta$. [+10.00D (−) +6.50D]

DISSIMILAR BIFOCAL SEGMENTS

The use of dissimilar segments with varying optical centers is a method for correcting vertical imbalance in a bifocal prescription. There are two possibilities. One involves the use of R-compensated segments. These designs were originated by Univis, Inc., and are currently available from

Vision-Ease (in glass only). The other involves different size Ultex-type, one-piece bifocals. Although these techniques have been made obsolete by slab-off grinding, the lenses are discussed here, not as recommended corrections but because a few geriatric patients having worn R-compensating segments for decades cling to the former method, and the latter is an accepted procedure in some parts of the world.

Vertical imbalance is eliminated or decreased by selecting two proper correcting segments, one of which has a low optical center (base-up prism). To counteract unwanted prism at near, one style is placed before the right eye, the other before the left. The result is not cosmetically pleasing because the appearance of each bifocal differs drastically. It is unusual for more than 1½ prism diopters to be corrected by this method. Since patients rarely experience problems until the imbalance exceeds that amount, the use of dissimilar segments is only a partial correction but may be enough to alleviate symptoms.

R-compensating Segments

Univis, Inc. created the R series of compensating bifocals. They are now available from Vision-Ease (in glass only). Since each prescription is custom made, the horizontal can be ordered 28mm or 26mm wide. All segments, however, measure 14mm vertically. The series consist of seven segments, each designated by the number that corresponds to optical-center positioning. The range is from #4 to #10. The upper and lower limits of each bifocal are straight lines varying in length.

The #4 has an optical center that is 4mm below the upper segment line, with the upper division longer than the lower (Figure 13.3).

In the #5 and #6 designs the upper line is also longer than the lower but not as long as the R #4 (Figures 13.4 and 13.5).

Since the #7 is the conventional R bifocal with the optical center halfway between, the top and bottom lines are equal (Figure 13.6).

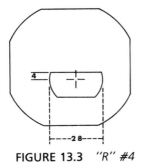

FIGURE 13.3 *"R" #4*

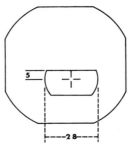

FIGURE 13.4 *"R" #5*

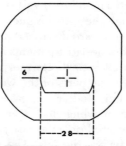

FIGURE 13.5   "R" #6

The #8 and #9 designs reverse the pattern with the lower line longer than the upper (Figures 13.7 and 13.8). The lower line reaches its maximum length in the R #10 design (Figure 13.9).

When compensating for vertical imbalance, the segment with the lowest optical center (for its base-down effect) is placed over the lens having the higher plus power.

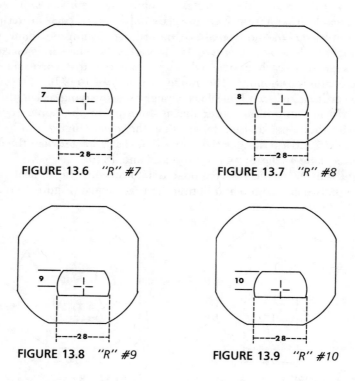

FIGURE 13.6   "R" #7   **FIGURE 13.7   "R" #8**

FIGURE 13.8   "R" #9   **FIGURE 13.9   "R" #10**

PROBLEM:

Given the following prescription:

O.D. $+1.00 -1.00 \times 45°$
O.S. $-1.00 -1.00 \times 30°$
O.U. Add $+3.00D$

The patient reads 8mm below the distance optical centers. Which of the lenses in the R-compensated series would correct the vertical imbalance?

PROCEDURE:

1. Determine the power in the meridian of each lens.

O.D. $+1.00 +(\frac{1}{2})(-1.00) = +0.50D$
O.S. $-1.00 +(\frac{3}{4})(-1.00) = -1.75D$

2. Determine the vertical imbalance.

$$V.I. = (+.50 - 1.75)(0.8)$$
$$= 1.8^{\Delta}$$

3. Compute the separation of the segment optical centers necessary to compensate for the vertical imbalance.

$$x = \frac{V.I.}{Add}$$
$$= \frac{1.8}{3.00}$$
$$= 0.6cm = 6mm$$

SOLUTION:

The following combination will correct the vertical imbalance:

O.D. R-compensating segment #10
O.S. R-compensating segment #4

Ultex-style One-piece Round-top Bifocals

The other method of compensating for vertical imbalance using dissimilar segments involves prescribing two different size Ultex-style one-piece, round-top bifocals. This method is not used in the United States. While the conventional Ultex E is no longer available here, it is available in other parts of the world.

There are four available lens designs in this series (the term "Ultex" is retained by common usage):

> Ultex B—O.C. 11mm down from the dividing line
>
> Ultex E—O.C. 16mm down from the dividing line
>
> Ultex A—O.C. 19 mm down from the dividing line
>
> Kingsize Ultex—O.C. 20mm down from the dividing line

PROBLEM:

Given the following prescription:

$$O.D. \ -2.00 \ -1.00 \times 30°$$
$$O.S. \ -0.50 \ -0.50 \times 45°$$
$$O.U. \ \text{Add} \ +3.00D$$

The patient reads 8mm below the distance optical center. Compensate for the vertical imbalance using Ultex one-piece round-top segments.

PROCEDURE:

1. Determine the power in the vertical meridian of each lens.

$$O.D. \ -2.00 \ +(\tfrac{3}{4}) \ (-1.00) = -2.75D$$
$$O.S. \ -0.50 \ +(\tfrac{1}{2}) \ (-0.50) = -0.75D$$

2. Determine the vertical imbalance.

$$V.I. = [-2.75 - (-0.75)] \ (0.8)$$
$$= 1.6^{\Delta}$$

3. Compute the separation of the segment optical centers necessary to compensate for the vertical imbalance.

$$x = \frac{V.I.}{\text{Add}}$$

$$= \frac{1.6}{3.00}$$

$$= 0.5 \text{ cm} = 5\text{mm separation}$$

SOLUTION:

The following lenses will correct the vertical imbalance:

> O.D. Ultex B (O.C. 11mm down from top of segment)
>
> O.S. Ultex E (O.C. 16mm down from top of segment)

PRISM SEGMENTS

Prism segments should never be used to correct vertical imbalance (counteracting imbalance by prism ground into the segments). This method is highly impractical for several reasons. Prism segments are most unattractive; there is pronounced distortion when the patient looks through the segments; the prism limits the near field of view. The procedure is mentioned here only to acquaint the reader with the disadvantages because it is described in publications involving compensations for vertical imbalance. The following example is given for clarity in understanding how it works and must not be construed as an example of how to prescribe. In fact, it is unlikely that segments with prism base-up/base-down are available in the United States. They are made in Europe. The last designs here with these possibilities were Panoptik prism segments manufactured by Bausch & Lomb, Inc., who have discontinued production of all prescription ophthalmic lenses.

PROBLEM:

Given the following prescription:

$$O.D. \ +4.00 \ D.S.$$
$$O.S. \ +2.00 \ D.S.$$
$$O.U. \ Add \ +2.00D$$

The patient reads 7mm below the distance optical centers. Compensate for the vertical imbalance at the near point using prism segments.

PROCEDURE:

1. Determine the amount of vertical imbalance.

$$V.I. = (4.00 - 2.00)(0.7)$$
$$= 1.4^\Delta$$

2. Therefore compensation is for 1^Δ (rounded off to the lowest $\frac{1}{2}^\Delta$).

SOLUTION:

$\frac{1}{2}^\Delta$ BD over O.D.; $\frac{1}{2}^\Delta$ BU over O.S. (divided equally between the two lenses).

Obviously, this problem serves only as an illustration; in any case, the amount of vertical imbalance is too small for a necessary compensation.

Chapter 14

PRESCRIPTION CHANGES INDUCED BY LENS TILT

INTRODUCTION

Modern frames are manufactured or fit so that the lower edges are angled in toward the cheeks. Positioning the glasses thus allows the eyewear to closely follow facial lines. (The term "glasses" continues from common usage.)

The angle between the vertical plane of the face and the positioning of the glasses, normally between 5 and 10°, is known as the pantoscopic tilt or pantoscopic angle.

Note: Theoretically, a retroscopic angle is one in which the lower edges of the frame are angled away from the vertical plane of the face. However, an actual retroscopic tilt is not used in the fitting of eyewear. The term is used clinically to designate a decrease in the pantoscopic angle.

CHANGE IN EFFECTIVE POWER

When a patient looks away from the optical center of a lens, an aberration known as oblique or marginal astigmatism is induced. Manufacturers of quality lenses usually correct this aberration for a line of sight passing 30° away from the optical center of the lens. However, as a result of the pantoscopic tilt, the correction for marginal astigmatism is nullified when the patient looks below the optical center.

If the lens power is low, the change in effective power is insignificant. When a higher power is involved, the pantoscopic angle may result in a prescription change critical to the patient.

When a spherical lens is tilted, two changes take place. The result is a new spherical power and the introduction of a cylinder power the axis of which is in the meridian of rotation. Since a pantoscopic angle is a tilt in the horizontal meridian, the resultant axis is 180°.

If a sphero-cylinder lens is tilted pantoscopically, the result is a new spherical power and a different cylinder power.

POWER CHANGES WHEN A PANTOSCOPIC TILT IS INVOLVED

When a lens is tilted pantoscopically, the change in power depends on two factors:

1.   The power of the lens in the vertical meridian.
2.   The angle of the tilt.

As the lens power and/or the angle increases, there is a greater increase in the power change. Two formulas describe the power variation: The first determines change in the spherical correction; the second determines the amount of induced cylinder.

$$F_{\text{new sphere}} = F_{\text{original sphere}} (1 + \tfrac{1}{3} \sin^2 \theta)$$

θ is the angle of tilt from the vertical plane

$$F_{\text{induced cylinder}} = F_{\text{original sphere}} (\tan^2 \theta)$$

The induced cylinder has the same sign as the power in the meridian involved. A plus sphere induces a plus cylinder while a minus sphere results in the introduction of a minus cylinder. Since the axis of the induced cylinder is in the meridian of rotation, it is 180°.

PROBLEM:

A +3.00D sphere is tilted pantoscopically 20°. What is the resultant prescription?

PROCEDURE:

1. Determine power of the new sphere.

$$F_{n.s.} = F_{o.s.} (1 + \tfrac{1}{3} \sin^2 \theta)$$
$$= +3.00(1 + \tfrac{1}{3} \sin^2 20°)$$
$$= +3.117D$$

2. Determine power of the induced cylinder.

$$F_{i.c.} = F_{o.s.}(\tan^2 \theta)$$
$$= +3.00(\tan^2 20°)$$
$$= +0.396D$$

3. Combine (1) and (2).

SOLUTION:

$+3.117D + 0.396D \times 180°$

PROBLEM:

A $-4.00D$ sphere is angled pantoscopically 15°. Find the new effective power.

PROCEDURE:

1. Determine the power of the new sphere.

$$F_{n.s.} = F_{o.s.}(1 + \tfrac{1}{3} \sin^2 \theta)$$
$$= -4.00(1 + \tfrac{1}{3} \sin^2 15°)$$
$$= -4.088D$$

2. Determine the power of the induced cylinder.

$$F_{i.c.} = F_{o.s.}(\tan^2 \theta)$$
$$= -4.00(\tan^2 15°)$$
$$= -0.288D$$

3. Combine (1) and (2).

SOLUTION:

$-4.088D - 0.288D \times 180°$

The above problems show only a small prescription change. Although there is a large angle of tilt, the lens powers are not high.

PROBLEM:

A $+7.00D$ sphere is angled pantoscopically 15°. Find the new effective power.

PROCEDURE:

1.   Determine the power of the new sphere.

$$F_{n.s.} = F_{o.s.}(1 + \tfrac{1}{3} \sin^2 \theta)$$
$$= +7.00(1 + \tfrac{1}{3} \sin^2 15°)$$
$$= +7.154D$$

2.   Determine the power of the induced cylinder.

$$F_{i.c.} = F_{o.s.}(\tan^2 \theta)$$
$$= +7.00(\tan^2 15°)$$
$$= +0.504D$$

3.   Combine (1) and (2).

SOLUTION:

$+7.154D + 0.504D \times 180°$

PROBLEM:

A $-6.00D$ sphere is tilted pantoscopically 20°. What is the new effective power?

PROCEDURE:

1.   Determine the power of the new sphere.

$$F_{n.s.} = F_{o.s.}(1 + \tfrac{1}{3} \sin^2 \theta)$$
$$= -6.00(1 + \tfrac{1}{3} \sin^2 20°)$$
$$= -6.234D$$

2.   Determine the power of the induced cylinder.

$$F_{i.c.} = F_{o.s.}(\tan^2 \theta)$$
$$= -6.00(\tan^2 20°)$$
$$= -0.792D$$

3.   Combine (1) and (2).

SOLUTION:

$-6.234D - 0.792D \times 180°$

The above two problems show a prescription change that may be significant to the patient.

PROBLEM:

A lens of $+14.00D$ is tilted pantoscopically 20°. What is the resultant effective power?

PROCEDURE:

1. Determine the power of the new sphere.

$$F_{n.s.} = F_{o.s.}(1 + \tfrac{1}{3}\sin^2 \theta)$$
$$= +14.00(1 + \tfrac{1}{3}\sin^2 20°)$$
$$= +14.566D$$

2. Determine the power of the induced cylinder.

$$F_{i.c.} = F_{o.s.}(\tan^2 \theta)$$
$$= +14.00(\tan^2 20°)$$
$$= +1.848D$$

3. Combine (1) and (2).

SOLUTION:

$+14.566D + 1.848D \times 180°$

This problem demonstrates that a high-power lens having a large pantoscopic tilt results in a prescription change that can be disturbing to the patient.

TILTING OF SPHERO-CYLINDER CORRECTIONS

If the original prescription includes a cylinder, only the total power in the vertical meridian is affected by the pantoscopic tilt. The power in the vertical meridian, therefore, is used to calculate the newly induced sphere and cylinder.

To determine the final effective power, the original cylinder is combined with the induced changes, as illustrated in the following examples.

PROBLEM:

A lens of $+5.00 - 1.00 \times 90°$ is tilted pantoscopically 15°. What is the resultant effective power?

PROCEDURE:

Since the cylinder axis is 90°, the total cylinder power is in the 180° meridian. Therefore, the cylinder in this example does not effect the total power in the vertical meridian.

1. Determine the power of the new sphere.

$$F_{n.s.} = F_{o.s.}(1 + \tfrac{1}{3}\sin^2 \theta)$$
$$= +5.00(1 + \tfrac{1}{3}\sin^2 15°)$$
$$= +5.11D$$

2.   Determine the power of the induced cylinder.

$$F_{i.c.} = F_{o.s.}(\tan^2 \theta)$$
$$= +5.00(\tan^2 15°)$$
$$= +0.36D$$

3.   The induced power is $+5.11 + 0.36 \times 180°$; transposed it is $+5.47 - 0.36 \times 90°$.

4.   Combine with original cylinder.

$$
\begin{array}{r}
+5.47 - 0.36 \times 90° \\
- 1.00 \times 90° \\
\hline
+5.47 - 1.36 \times 90°
\end{array}
$$

SOLUTION:

$+5.47D - 1.36D \times 90°$

PROBLEM:

A lens of $-3.00 + 1.00 \times 180°$ is tilted pantoscopically 20°. What is the effective power?

PROCEDURE:

Since the cylinder axis is 180°, the total power of the cylinder is in the vertical meridian. By transposing the lens formula $-3.00 +1.00 \times 180°$ to $-2.00-1.00 \times 90°$ it is seen that the power in the vertical meridian is $-2.00D$.

1.   Determine the power of the new sphere.

$$F_{n.s.} = F_{o.s.}(1 + \tfrac{1}{3} \sin^2 \theta)$$
$$= -2.00(1 + \tfrac{1}{3} \sin^2 20°)$$
$$= -2.078D$$

2.   Determine the power of the induced cylinder.

$$F_{i.c.} = F_{o.s.}(\tan^2 \theta)$$
$$= -2.00(\tan^2 20°)$$
$$= -0.264D$$

3.   The induced power is $-2.078 - 0.264 \times 180°$; transposed it is $-2.342 + 0.264 \times 90°$.

4. Combine with cylinder of the transposed form in the original problem.

$$
\begin{array}{r}
-1.00 \ \times 90° \\
\underline{-2.342 + 0.264 \times 90°} \\
-2.342 - 0.736 \times 90°
\end{array}
$$

SOLUTION:

+3.078D + 0.736D × 180° (in original form)

PRACTICAL CONSIDERATIONS

The problems were given to demonstrate the effect of a pantoscopic angle. From a practical viewpoint computations are usually not necessary when determining a prescription. The high correction is placed in a trial frame, which is adjusted at the spectacle plane. The practitioner then refines to give the best visual acuity before writing the final prescription.

WRAP-AROUND FRAME DESIGNS

Wrap-around, goggle-type frame designs result in a distortion similar to that of the pantoscopic tilt. However, the problem of distortion is more acute because these frames are designed with a wrap-around angle as high as 35°. The resultant longitudinal peripheral distortion can be intolerable to the patient.

The formulas demonstrating the power change in wrap-around eyewear are the same as those involved in the pantoscopic tilt except for the following change. Since the lenses are tilted about the vertical axis, the power in the horizontal meridian is affected; therefore, the induced cylinder is axis 90°.

PROBLEM:

The patient wears a prescription O.U. +4.00 −0.50 × 90°. If the correction is duplicated in a goggle-type sunframe that angles toward the face 15°, what is the resultant effective power?

PROCEDURE:

1. Transpose to determine the power at 180°.

$$+3.50 + 0.50 \times 180°$$

2. Determine the power of the new sphere.

$$F_{n.s.} = F_{o.s.}(1 + \tfrac{1}{3} \sin^2 \theta)$$
$$= +3.50(1 + \tfrac{1}{3} \sin^2 15°)$$
$$= +3.577D$$

3. Determine the power of the induced cylinder.

$$F_{i.c.} = F_{o.s.}(\tan^2 \theta)$$
$$= +3.50(\tan^2 15°)$$
$$= +0.252D$$

4. Induced power $= +3.577 + 0.252 \times 90°$

Transpose and combine with cylinder from step (1)

$$+3.829 - 0.252 \times 180°$$
$$\underline{ + 0.50 \ \times 180°}$$
$$+3.829 + 0.248 \times 180°$$

SOLUTION:

$+4.077 - 0.248 \times 90°$ (in original form)

PROBLEM:

A lens of $-5.00 + 1.00 \times 180°$ is duplicated in a wrap-around frame tilted 25° toward the temples. What is the resultant effective power?

PROCEDURE:

1. Determine the power of the new sphere.

$$F_{n.s.} = F_{o.s.}(1 + \tfrac{1}{3} \sin^2 \theta)$$
$$= -5.00(1 + \tfrac{1}{3} \sin^2 25°)$$
$$= -5.30D$$

2. Determine the power of the induced cylinder.

$$F_{i.c.} = F_{o.s.} (\tan^2 \theta)$$
$$= -5.00(\tan^2 25°)$$
$$= +1.085D$$

3. Induced power $= -5.30 - 1.085 \times 90°$

4. Transpose induced power to axis 180°.

$$-6.385 + 1.085 \times 180°$$

5.   Combine with original cylinder.

$$-6.385 + 1.085 \times 180°$$
$$+ 1.00 \ \times 180°$$
$$\overline{-6.385 + 2.085 \times 180°}$$

SOLUTION:

$-6.385 + 2.085 \times 180°$

The above example clearly shows that the prescription change caused by angling of a lens can be disturbing to the patient.

Sensitivity to the wrap-around angle when low-power lenses are involved varies with the individual. Some patients find almost any horizontal distortion intolerable, particularly when operating a motor vehicle; others will ignore the aberration if the amount is not too great. Fortunately, the problem has been lessened with the current availability of great numbers of chic sunframes that are not curved toward the temples.

LENS DESIGNS AND CONTEMPORARY EYE FRAMES

INTRODUCTION

The wide variety of materials used in the manufacture of contemporary eyewear has made possible the greatest choice of frame fashions in history. Almost every basic design of every era has been expanded to meet modern styling needs ranging from the conventional to the avant-garde. The majority of frames are made of plastic; a relative few are made of aluminum or nylon. Others are fashioned of metal, gold, or gold-filled wires. Some feature more than one kind of material on a single-frame fashion. Often certain types of lenses offer definite advantages when used in conjunction with specific frame types. This chapter includes a discussion of contemporary stylings with recommendations about lenses providing the best service to the patient.

PLASTIC FRAMES

Frames fashioned of zylonite (cellulose acetate) and optyl plastic are the most popular of the contemporary designs. These materials are often the choice of famous designers because they lend themselves admirably to the beauty of haute couture.

Optyl, introduced in Europe during the late 1960s, has been marketed extensively in the United States for the past decade. In many ways it is a remarkable material. Optyl retains its beauty almost indefinitely; it is not affected by exposure to the elements, such as sun and wind. Secretions of the skin—perspiration or oil—do not change its appearance; neither does hair spray. Therefore, the grayish films that often form on zylonite frames, particularly along the temples, are absent. Unlike other frame materials, it is hypoallergenic; there has not been a single case on record of a skin rash resulting from optyl mountings. It is comfortable to wear, weighing about one-third less than a comparable zylonite frame. Once adjusted, it keeps its alignment indefinitely unless reheated, whereby it goes back to its original factory shape (it has complete memory). CR 39 lenses have less bitoric effect when used with optyl than with other frame materials. In every tested sampling the eyewear conforms to ANSI standards for ophthalmic prescriptions.

Although the current fashion look in eyewear spotlights the small designs, there are patients who prefer larger mountings, particularly for sunwear. Plastic frames with a rigid pad bridge construction, particularly the optyl designs, when coupled with CR 39 or polycarbonate lenses offer the ultimate in comfort. Such frames can work with glass lenses to provide comfortable eyewear, although glass sometimes presents weight problems, particularly with high-index designs and some photochromic lenses.

Contemporary fashion emphasizes tinted lenses. CR 39 lenses tint beautifully into any color and will give any desired effect. Some manufacturers supply clear, tintable plastic frames, so lenses and frame can be made the same color. This custom look is especially enjoyed because it can obviously be a one-of-a-kind fashion.

Plastic frames result in the best cosmetic look for high minus and prism corrections because the rims cover much of the edges. The hide-a-bevel method of finishing these lenses should always be used. When tinted a hue in the same color family as the primary shade of the frame to eliminate the sharp line of demarcation between lenses and mounting, the cosmetic effect is the best possible.

METAL AND GOLD-FILLED MOUNTINGS (WIRES)

In the 1940s through the middle 1950s frames featuring metal rims surrounding the lenses were dispensed almost exclusively to industrial workers whose occupations made durability a prime concern. In the late 1950s and early 1960s these industrial frames were replaced largely by plastic designs because most workers during that period preferred their cosmetic appeal. In addition, since industrial-thickness glass lenses were almost always prescribed, plastic frames resulted in more comfortable eyewear. Metal mountings had adjustable pad bridge designs, and these small contact areas carrying most of the weight of the glasses often left sore marks on the nose.

A dramatic reappearance of these metal frames took place about the middle to late 1960s. Spurred by the hippie movement, many teenagers and young college students sought these obsolete styles in shops specializing in "elegant junk," bringing the styles into professional offices for lens prescriptions. Optical manufacturers, recognizing marketing potential, added a touch of fashion to the basic designs and introduced narrow "granny" wires. The popularity of metal frames is still here, with current designs featuring both the narrow-look and mountings having a deep vertical dimension.

Some of the newer metal mountings are constructed with a plastic bridge, but the majority have an adjustable pad bridge construction. When glass lenses are mounted into the latter, patients frequently complain of nasal pressure as well as unsightly red marks on the nose. Sometimes the complaints are severe, especially if the lenses are oversize, thicker than conventional (i.e., photochromics or high-power corrections) or if the patient has undergone rhinoplasty (nose surgery). Plastic lenses are the most satisfactory choice for wire frames.

In cases of high minus or prism corrections, wirelike frames may not be cosmetically suitable, because the edges are almost completely exposed. If the patient insists on a metal mounting, the problem can be minimized when the hide-a-bevel method of finishing the lenses is used.

The use of a light tint enhances the fashion value of eyewear for general wear because it "covers" the whitish bevel common to hard-resin lenses. The hues that look best while keeping the visible spectrum relatively intact are pale pinks, soft grays, and very light tans. Some practitioners order polished lens edges for cosmetic value, but availability is often a problem because not all optical laboratories provide this service. Some patients do not like the look.

It is sometimes tempting to recommend high-index glass for the high myopic patient who insists on a wire mounting. This is rarely a satisfactory procedure. Although the lenses are relatively thin, they are comparatively heavy. This is especially annoying if the mounting is a large-eye fashion and has an adjustable pad bridge construction. (The use of the brittle flint glass, Thinlite, in single-vision and one-piece multifocal lenses was eliminated with the FDA ruling regarding impact-resistant lenses. The new high-index glass, distributed under various trade names, can be chemically tempered. The local laboratory should be queried for prescription availability.) Polycarbonate lenses are the best choice. Although not quite as thin as high-index glass, they have excellent cosmetic value and can be tinted many beautiful shades.

COMBINATION AND COMBINATION-TYPE MOUNTINGS

An amazing development is the emerging of combination and combination-type frames into the world of fashion eyewear. The former are "factory worker" mountings issued since the 1940s; the latter have been primarily an "older person" mounting, especially for the low-vision patient. Both designs are characterized by metal rims (called a chassis) circling the lenses. Combination mountings are topped by wide zylonite bars and usually have zylonite temples. Combination-type frames feature aluminum tops/temples. Both are "small" eye fashions, almost always with 52mm as the largest available eye size. The bridges have an adjustable pad construction.

In 1986 these frames began appearing on the faces of theatrical personalities who set fashion trends. Almost always, the lenses are deeply tinted and/or "mirrored." Evolving as important contemporary fashions in the late 1980s, the trend will undoubtedly continue into the 1990s. Mirrored lenses tend to be best in glass form (the small sizes rarely make weight a problem even with the adjustable pad bridge) since mirror coatings have been known to "peel" from CR 39 lenses. However, that problem should be solved in the near future. Recently the lenses have been seen in pretty, soft shadings like rose and soft blue. For these solid and gradient tints, plastic lenses are the best recommendation.

RIMLESS DESIGNS

In the 1930s and 1940s the most popular frames were rimless-type mountings. Lens edges were completely exposed. Most featured a bar (sometimes called an arm) that curved upward from the bridge to follow along and behind the upper edges of the lens. Others were what manufacturers call a "complete rimless"; the bar was absent and so the lenses were attached to the mounting at four points (two nasal and two temporal). In the 1950s they were replaced by plastic frames and it became rare to see patients wearing rimless designs. In the 1960s the hippie movement brought rimless along with wire mountings back into fashion. Their popularity has continued to this day, and succeeding decades have spotlighted consistently updated, elegant versions.

Plastic lenses serve particularly well in rimless designs. In fact, some laboratories will not fill prescriptions asking for drilled glass lenses, which readily break at the points of attachment. Patients sometimes request unusual shapes (resembling hearts, flowers, etc.), and CR 39 plastic can be hand-formed easily to almost any desired pattern.

When high minus lenses or prism corrections are involved, the appearance of the exposed thick edges can present a problem. If cosmetic value is critical, it may be best to recommend a frame design that covers the bevels, although controlling the lens size is a possible answer. As a guide, a −4.00D hard-resin CR 39 lens having a 54mm horizontal box measurement will be about 6 mm thick on the temporal edges.

The most popular rimless designs today are the "nylon-suspension" frames. These feature a clear nylon thread that circles the lenses. Breakage is almost impossible because the lenses are not drilled, and glass designs, such as photochromics, can be used if desired. However, there are problems with some bevels, and certain lens designs may not stay in place, e.g., laminated lenses. If in doubt, query the laboratory.

For maximum esthetic appeal, lenses in a rimless frame should be fashion tinted. Some of the color effects, such as gradient tints and two tones in juxtaposition, are easily achieved with CR 39 lenses and are stunning on deep-shaped patterns. The range in tint possibilities for polycarbonates is expanding and should match that of hard-resin plastic in the very near future.

Complete rimless mountings are almost always the choice of patients desiring jeweling on a lens, since the absence of rims focuses attention on the design. The lenses must be CR 39. The jewels should be small in size and placed on the lower temporal corner of one lens so as not to interfere with vision. Tinted lenses should serve as the fashion background. In the 1970s this effect was extremely popular, particularly the personalized jeweled initials, but the 1980s showed a slowdown in requests. Contemporary fashions tend to be complete rimless designs with a deep color on the edges of softly tinted CR 39 lenses, usually in the same color family, e.g., pink lenses, with deep rose circling the bevels.

ALUMINUM FRAMES

Full-size aluminum frames are rarely dispensed today, but interestingly, half-eye aluminum mountings are very much in demand. The gold and silver-appearing designs look like elegant jewelry and those in fashion colors lend themselves to a marvelous avant-garde look. Some wearers prefer glass lenses for half-eye mountings because of the frequent taking-off/putting-on process. However, aluminum is a rigid metal and hard-resin lenses usually insure that the edges will not chip. While a full-size aluminum frame is not necessarily heavier than a plastic design, it is seldom as comfortable. This probably results from the feeling of metal against the skin. The patient is best served when plastic lenses are recommended.

NYLON FRAMES

The allure of nylon frames is that they are almost indestructible under certain conditions. Yet there are a number of considerations that limit their use. Although the frame colors have been improved drastically, they rarely meet the beauty possibilities of zylonite plastic, the material they most resemble visually. Nylon is difficult to adjust with conventional frame-heating devices. (Manufacturers recommend using hot water.) In very cold weather it may become brittle and crack. The solution according to manufacturers is immersing the eyewear in water overnight several times a week so that dehydration does not take place. Obviously, this is not always convenient.

There is a special nylon sport frame having a rubberized nose/bridge area and riding-bow temples that, when held on the head with an athletic strap hooked through the temples, proves highly efficient for the patient engaged in contact sports. For safety's sake, plastic lenses should be mounted in this design. While nylon clamps down on hard-resin prescription lenses creating a relatively high bitoric effect, the eyewear, limited to sporting activities, is rarely worn long enough to give rise to aesthenopia.

Note: In all testing of CR 39 prescription lenses mounted into nylon frames, the bitoric effect was too high to meet the standards set by ANSI.

A number of manufacturers are making available nylon frames with plano polycarbonate lenses for use as active-wear fashions. These are the safest form of eyewear available and make the best use of nylon frames.

HALF-EYE FRAMES

Half-eye frames are used as reading prescription eyewear. Designed to be small—usually a 46, 48, or 50mm eyesize—they are worn low on the nose, enabling the patient to look over them for distant viewing. Contemporary half-eyes are available in aluminum, plastic, nylon, metal (wire), and rimless styles. Glass can be the lens of choice because half-eyes are often subjected to the taking-off/putting-on process, making a highly scratch-resistant lens the most practical. Weight should not present a problem since the frame is small and the correction is rarely greater than +2.50D. When the half-eye frame is fashioned of aluminum or metal or is a drilled rimless mounting, plastic lenses should be seriously considered, because edge chipping is a consideration. Coatings that make the front surface of CR 39 as scratch-resistant as glass are easily available. Quality polycarbonate lenses have factory-placed coatings that make them very practical.

LORGNETTES

Lorgnettes are meant to be held before the eyes when a presbyope needs momentary clear vision. They are usually fashioned of plastic or gold-filled metal. When not in use, most fold at the bridge, with the lenses slipping into the hollow handle that is part of the design. They are used primarily by women who display them as styled accessories, e.g., while reading a dinner menu, glancing at a theater program, etc.

Lenses mounted into a lorgnette frame must be ground with flat base curves if they are to fit properly into the handle. Glass is the only suitable design because it is difficult, if not impossible, to order the desired curvature in plastic lenses.

It may be practical to recommend lorgnette frames with lenses already mounted into them. A few optical concerns stock them with glass lenses of powers +1.50D spheres, +2.00D spheres, and +2.50D spheres. It is rarely necessary to order the patient's exact near correction because the eyewear is used only minutes at a time.

FRAME CONSIDERATIONS IN MULTIFOCAL PRESCRIBING

It is always a concern when frame fashions concentrate on a narrow-appearing design (difference of 10mm or greater between the horizontal "A" and vertical "B" measurements) because there is difficulty in giving the multifocal patient a suitable near area. With such frames clinical experience reveals that wider segments should be ordered for compensation. If a flat-top segment is 13mm high, the horizontal bifocal measurement should be at least 28mm; if the trifocal is 19mm, a straight-top 7 × 28mm is the best for general wear.

Fortunately, contemporary eyeframes spotlight so many designs that deep lens shapes allowing for a higher segment are easily available. It is not unusual to order general-wear bifocals 19, 20, and 21mm high (the segment line positioned just below or at the lower lid for easy neck and head posturing). The intermediate segment in a trifocal is customarily 7mm in depth, so an overall height of 22mm—usually the intermediate line is about 1mm below the lower pupil margin in normal indoor illumination—allows for a comfortable 15mm-high near segment.

When prescribing seamless (blended) bifocals, it is important to use a frame with a deep vertical dimension. The blur circle that separates the distance from the near correction is easier to ignore when the ordered segment height is at least 20mm.

Although progressive addition lenses must be inserted into a frame allowing a minimum of 22mm from the pupil center to the lower lens edge (see Chapter 5, "Prescribing 'Invisible' Multifocals"), a mounting that provides a longer measurement is more satisfactory, because it gives the patient a larger near field.

All occupational multifocals require frames with a deep vertical dimension allowing for the necessary high segment positioning. Fortunately, such designs are frequently available with adjustable pads that allow the lenses to be set precisely for better patient satisfaction.

BIBLIOGRAPHY

Atchison, D.A., Laboratory evaluation of commercial aspheric aphakic lenses, Am. J. Optom., 60 (7): 598, 1983.

Atchison, D.A., Third-order theory and aspheric spectacle lens design, Ophthal. Physiol. Opt., 4 (2): 179, 1984.

Atchison, D.A., Spectacle lens design, development and present state, Australian J. Optom., 67 (3): 97, 1984.

Atchison, D.A., Clinical trial with commercial aspheric aphakic lenses, Am. J. Optom., 61 (9): 566, 1984.

Atchison, D.A., Modern optical design assessment and spectacle lenses, Optica. Acta., 32 (5): 607, 1985.

Bailey, I.L., Equivalent viewing power or magnification, which is fundamental?, Optician, 188 (4970): 32, 1984.

Barth, R., New aspherical lens for aphakia, Optician, 185 (4780): 22, 1983.

Bennett, I., The changing world of lenses, Optometric Management, 19 (9): 29, 1983.

Bennett, I., Guarantee against scratches, Optometric Management, 22 (11): 60, 1986.

Bennett, A.G., Two simple calculating schemes for use in ophthalmic optics, I. Tracing oblique rays through systems . . . , Ophthal. Physiol. Opt., 6 (3): 325, 1986.

Bennett, A.G., Two simple calculating schemes for use in ophthalmic optics, II. Tracing axial pencils through systems . . . , Ophthal. Physiol. Opt., 6 (4): 419, 1986.

Berry, E.A., An evaluation of lenses designed to block light emitted by light-curing units, J. Am. Dental Assoc., 112 (1): 70, 1986.

Blumlein, S.J., The technical merits of modern lenses, Optician, 192 (5056): 28, 1986.

Bonsett-Veal, J.D., Enhancing the cosmetic appearance of high minus spectacle lenses, Optom. Monthly, 75 (1): 12, 1984.

Borish, I.M., Aphakia, perceptual and refractive problems of spectacle correction, J. Am. Optom. Assoc., 54 (8): 701, 1983.

Chaudri, M.M., The catastrophic failure of thermally tempered glass caused by small-particle impact, Nature, 320 (6057): 48, 1986.

Chou, B.R., Reflections on anti-reflection coatings, Canadian J. Optom., 45 (1): 30, 1983.

Chou, B.R., Spectral transmittance of selected tinted ophthalmic lenses, Canadian J. Optom., 45 (4): 192, 1983.

Chou, B.R., Spectral characteristics of sports and occupational tinted lenses, Canadian J. Optom., 47 (2): 77, 1985.

Chou, B.R., Optical radiation protection by non-prescription sunglasses, Canadian J. Optom., 48 (1): 17, 1986.

Clark, B.A.J., Near infrared absorption in sunglasses, Australian J. Optom., 65 (5): 192, 1982.

Corth, R., The perception of depth contours with yellow goggles, an alternative explanation, Perception, 14 (3): 377, 1985.

Coulon, M., Evaluating the scratch-resistance of organic lenses, Optical World, 14 (89): 8, 1985.

Davey, G.V., Polycarbonate, the everyday lens, Optical World, 13 (79): 44, 1984.

Davey, G.V., Polycarbonate, high hopes for high myopes, Dispensing Optician, 36 (4): 223, 1984.

Davey, J.B., Tinted motorcyclists' visors, Manufacturing Optics International, 35 (8): 11, 1982.

Davey, J.B., Sunglasses from opticians, optical quality and additional protection, Ophthal. Opt., 29 (3): 64, 1983.

Davey, J.B., Slimline, CPL adds to the high index range, Ophthal. Opt., 23 (10): 318, 1983.

Davey, J.B., Photochromic glass, Pilkingtons world-wide success benefit UKS RX market, Optical World, 12 (78): 7, 1984.

Davey, J.B., Uses of light photochromatic glasses, Optician, 187 (4930): 14, 1984.

Davey, J.B., Surface coatings were never better, Optician, 187 (4935): 12, 1984.

Davey, J.B., Coating and caution, Optician, 189 (4986): 25, 1985.

Davey, J.B., At last, impact-resistant spectacles, Optician, 189 (4999): 13, 1985.

Davey, J.B., Tints, sunspectacles and standards, update on lens material for sunglasses, Optician, 191 (5030): 24, 1986.

Davey, J.B., Tints and cosmetic coatings, Optician, 193 (5080): 18, 1987.

Davis, J.K., The properties of lenses used for the correction of aphakia, J. Am. Optom. Assoc., 54 (8): 685, 1983.

De Faria E Sousa, S.J., HP program for the center thickness of convex spectacle lenses, Am. J. Optom., 63 (9): 770, 1986.

De Lucas, L.J., How to estimate the edge thickness of a minus lens, South. J. Optom., 1 (3): 21, 1983.

Drew, R., A new lens material, the best of two worlds, Corning's bond of glass and plastic . . . , Optical Management, 11 (6): 13, 1982.

Drew, R., High-index glass, the cosmetic trend, Optical Management, 12 (10): 20, 1983.

Drew, R., CR 39 slab-off lenses, now ready cast, Optical Management, 13 (1): 21, 1984.

Duckworth, W.H., Strength of glass lenses processed in an ultrasonically stimulated chem-tempering bath, Am. J. Optom., 61 (1): 48, 1984.

Enoch, J.M., Helping the aphakic neonate to see, International Ophthalmology, 8 (4): 237, 1985.

Fowler, C.W., Aspheric lenses, Optician, 184 (4753): 14, 1982.

Fowler, C.W., Choosing and using aspheric spectacle lenses, Optician, 185 (4780): 13, 1983.

Fowler, C.W., Patents review, some recent patents on ophthalmic lenses, Ophthal. Physiol. Opt., 3 (2): 193, 1983.

Fowler, C.W., The Wrobel Super-Lenti, a new lens for the high myope, Optician, 185 (4796): 26, 1983.

Fowler, C.W., Aspheric spectacle lens designs for aphakia, Am. J. Optom., 61 (12): 737, 1984.

Fowler, C.W., Two spectacle lenses for aphakia, Ophthal. Physiol. Opt., 4 (4): 369, 1984.

Fowler, C.W., Aspheric lenses, present and future, Optician, 189 (4977): 11, 1985.

Fowler, C.W., Some notes on the construction of zonal aspheric aphakic spectacle lenses, Ophthal. Physiol. Opt., 5 (3): 343, 1985.

Fowler, C.W., Questions and answers on aspheric lenses, Optician, 191 (5028): 18, 1986.

Fowler, C.W., Progressive lens developments, Optician, 192 (5068): 28, 1986.

Freeman, M.B., Can you have a distance and near pd with an executive bifocal?, Optom. Mon., 75 (11): 449, 1984.

Freeman, M.B., Lenses of the future, Optician, 191 (5050): 23, 1986.

Giulino, G., Recent developments in ophthalmic lenses, Dispensing Optician, 36 (4): 214, 1984.

Goldsmith, W., Fracture characteristics of ophthalmic lenses, Am. J. Optom., 60 (11): 914, 1983.

Good, G.W., The use of progressive addition multifocals with video display terminals, J. Am. Optom. Assoc., 57 (9): 654, 1986.

Greenberg, I., Statistical protocol for impact testing prescription polycarbonate safety lenses, Optical World, 14 (85): 7, 1985.

Gruber, E., Keeping current on ophthalmic lenses, Ophthalmology Management, 2 (6): 26, 1984.

Harrison, W.R., Photochromic lenses, Optom. Today, 12 (3): 28, 1986.

Hellinger, G., Use of the CPF lenses for light sensitive individuals, J. Vis. Impair Blind, 77 (9): 449, 1983.

Hensley, L.E., The balance lens, an ophthalmic orphan, Optical Management, 11 (8): 25, 1982.

Hirschhorn, H., Polycarbonates, an urban report, Optical Management, 12 (5): 35, 1983.

Hirschhorn, H., Fresnel press-on optics, Optical Management, 13 (3): 41, 1984.

Hitzeman, S.A., Comparison of the acceptance of progressive addition multifocal vs. a standard multifocal lens design, J. Am. Optom. Assoc., 56 (9): 706, 1985.

Hoffman, L., Modified frame with CPF-lens gives enlarged field of view, Rec. Optom., 121 (9): 95, 1984.

Holle, M.R., Pros and cons of a Fresnel lens low vision aid, J. Am. Optom. Assoc., 56 (7): 566, 1985.

Honson, V.J., Resistance of transparent plastics to surface abrasion, Clin. Exp. Optom., 69 (1): 27, 1986.

Jalie, M., Practical ophthalmic lenses, plus lenses, back surface compensation, semi-finished sphere blanks, Manufacturing Optics International, 36 (6): 11, 1983.

Jalie, M., High refractive index glass lenses, Optician, 186 (4805): 10, 1983.

Jalie, M., Solid bifocals revisited, Optician, 189 (4984): 42, 1985.

Jalie, M., Prism-controlled solid bifocals, Optom. Today, 25 (13): 436, 1985.

Jalie, M., Recent lens developments, Dispensing Optics, 1 (3): 12, 1986.

Jones, W.F., High index now in crown glass, Optician, 186 (4821): 26, 1983.

Kalra, V.K., Optics of aphakia, Optom. Today, 12 (2): 53, 1986.

Keating, M.P., Dioptric power in an off meridian, the torsional component, Am. J. Optom., 63 (10): 830, 1986.

Kelly, S.A., Effect of yellow-tinted lenses on contrast sensitivity, Am. J. Optom., 61 (11): 657, 1984.

Kilum, D., Dispensing Varilux 2, tolerance of variation in threshold fitting heights GHTS, Dispensing Optics, 1 (3): 16, 1986.

Kinney, J.A.S., Reaction time to spatial frequencies using yellow and luminance-matched neutral goggles, Am. J. Optom., 60 (2): 132, 1983.

Krefman, R.A., Multiple coatings, Int. Eyecare, 1 (6): 410, 1985.

Kumar, N., Plastic lenses, Optom. Today, 12 (2): 27, 1986.

Le Texier, F., Generalization of the Tscherning theory, optimization of aspheric ophthalmic lenses, Ophthal. Physiol. Opt., 7 (1): 63, 1987.

Lovell, D.J., Commercially available computerized lens design programs, Laser Focus, 20 (8): 98, 1984.

Luria, S.M., Preferred density of sunglasses, Am. J. Optom., 61 (6): 397, 1984.

Lynch, D., An evaluation of the Corning CPF 550 lens, Optom. Mon., 75 (1): 36, 1984.

Magnante, D.B., Ultraviolet absorption of commonly used clip-on sunglasses, Annals of Ophthalmology, 17 (10): 614, 1985.

Margach, C.B., Executives, Optometric Extension Program, 58 (10): 71, 1986.

Megla, G.K., Selectively absorbing glasses for the potential prevention of ocular disorders, Applied Optics, 22 (8): 1216, 1983.

Morrissette, D.L., Users and nonusers evaluations of the CPF 550 lenses, Am. J. Optom., 61 (11): 704, 1984.

Mousa, G.Y., Control of glare for VDT operators, part 1: transmission of fluorescent light through UV filters and pink . . . , Can. J. Optom., 48 (1): 47, 1986.

Mousa, G.Y., Control of glare for VDT operators, evaluation of different lenses by subjects, Optovision, 48 (2): 77, 1986.

Mullins, P., The growing versatility of photochromic glass, South African Optometrist, 42 (2): 103, 1983.

Peli, E. Control of vertically polarized glare, J. Am. Optom. Assoc., 54 (5): 447, 1983.

Rosek, K., Premolded slab-offs bring results, Optical Management, 13 (8): 27, 1984.

Rosenthal, F.S., The effect of prescription eyewear on ocular exposure to ultraviolet radiation, Am. J. Public Health, 76 (10): 1216, 1986.

Saragas, S., Simple method for locating the optical center of a lens, Annals of Ophthalmology, 16 (5): 408, 1984.

Sasieni, L.S., Guide to high power lenses, Optician, 188 (4956): 7, 1984.

Saunders, H., The algebra of sphero-cylinders, Ophthal. Physiol. Opt., 5 (2): 157, 1985.

Scrivener, A.B., Developments in ophthalmic materials, Dispensing Optician, 35 (7): 198, 1983.

Sheedy, J.E., Optics of progressive addition lenses, Am. J. Optom., 64 (2): 90, 1987.

Shupnick, M., Finish first with finished multifocals, Opt. Index, 58 (6): 64, 1983.

Silver, J.H., Do retinitis pigmentosa patients prefer red photochromic lenses?, Ophthal. Physiol. Opt., 5 (1): 87, 1985.

Silver, J.H., Sunglasses, guidance for the optometrist, Optom. Today, 25 (19): 620, 1985.

Simonet, P., Peripheral power variations in progressive addition lenses, Am. J. Optom., 63 (11): 873, 1986.

Sliker, J., The impact of scratch-resistant coatings, Optical Management, 12 (6): 21, 1983.

Smith, G., Construction, specification, and mathematical description of aspheric surfaces, Am. J. Optom., 60 (3): 216, 1983.

Smith, G., Aspheric high positive power lenses and third order theory, Am. J. Optom., 60 (10): 843, 1983.

Smith, G., Aspheric surfaces and lenses in ophthalmic optics, Australian J. Optom., 68 (4): 125, 1985.

Spiegler, J.B., Lens weight as a function of density, shape and power, Am. J. Optom., 59 (8): 653, 1982.

Steer, L.M., The kitemark scheme for industrial eye protectors, Optician, 185 (4790): 17, 1983.

Sutton, A., Magnification-minification, characteristics of lenses and prisms, Optometric Extension Program, 57 (11): 35, 1985.

Tupper, B., The effect of a 550NM cutoff filter on the vision of cataract patients, Annals of Ophthalmology, 17 (1): 67, 1985.

Underwood, J., Prismatic effects in spectacle lenses, Optician, 188 (4970): 13, 1984.

Weber, H., Polycarbonate lens technology, Manufacturing Optics International, 36 (6): 22, 1983.

Wilkinson, P., Scratch resistance and optical properties of plastic lens coatings, Optician, 188 (4962): 18, 1984.

Wilkinson, P., The latest revision of the spectacle lens standard, part 1, Optician, 188 (4973): 28, 1984.

Wilkinson, P., The latest revision of the spectacle lens standard, part 2, Optician, 188 (4974): 40, 1984.

Wolfson, L., A modified quartz coating technique, Optical Management, 11 (8): 31, 1982.

Woodcock, F.R., Update on organic lenses, Optician, 186 (4822): 16, 1983.

Woodcock, F.R., High index lenses, Optician, 188 (4962): 23, 1984.

Woodcock, F.R., Vacuum coating machines, an update on new processes and equipment available, Optical World, 13 (83): 10, 1984.

Woodcock, F.R., Bifocal lens update, Optician, 189 (4995): 21, 1985.

Woodcock, F.R., Aspheric lenses for post-cataract wear, Optical World, 14 (90): 2, 1985.

Woodcock, F.R., An everchanging scene, upmarket multifocals, Optician, 192 (5064): 22, 1986.

Woodcock, F.R., Lens toughening by thermal process, Optical World, 15 (99): 18, 1986.

Woodcock, F.R., Chemical lens tempering, Optical World, 15 (100): 12, 1987.

Woodcock, F.R., Coating for organic lenses, Optom. Today, 27 (2): 37, 1987.

Yap, M., The effect of a yellow filter on contrast sensitivity, Ophthal. Physiol. Opt., 4 (3): 227, 1984.

Young, J.M., The photolite lens, a plastic photosensitive lens from AO, Optical World, 11 (72): 4, 1983.

INDEX